Ethics, Jurisprudence and History for the Dental Hygienist

Ethics,
Jurisprudence
and History

for the Dental Hygienist

WILMA E. MOTLEY, R.D.H.

Department of Dental Hygiene
University of Southern California School of Dentistry
Los Angeles, California

Second Edition

LEA & FEBIGER · *Philadelphia*

Library of Congress Cataloging in Publication Data

Motley, Wilma E
  Ethics, jurisprudence, and history for the dental hygienist.

  Includes bibliographical references and index.
  1. Dental hygienists. 2. Dental ethics. 3. Dental jurisprudence. 4. Dental hygiene—History. I. Title. [DNLM: 1. Dental hygienists. 2. Dental prophylaxis—History. 3. Ethics, Dental. 4. Forensic dentistry. WU50 M919e]
  RK60.5.M64   1975   174'.2   75-19242
  ISBN 0-8121-0529-X

First Edition, 1972

Published in Great Britain by Henry Kimpton Publishers, London

PRINTED IN THE UNITED STATES OF AMERICA

Print number: 3   2

Preface

There have been no textbooks on ethics for dental hygienists and comparatively few articles on the subject have been directed to this group. Therefore the major objectives of this book are to provide: appropriate factual background on the theory of the philosophy of ethics in a coherent, relevant form; an outline of situations provocative of serious thought on ethics; material on which classroom discussion on the practical application of ethics can be based. Jurisprudence for the dental hygienist and history of oral hygiene and the professional organization of dental hygiene are included as individual chapters.

Discourses on ethics, for use in today's world of permissiveness, might seem to represent wasted effort, yet they are essential to the moral growth of the individual. It is right that students should question and challenge philosophical ideas new to them or in conflict with their current concepts. The instructor who shares his perception with students and encourages a cooperative dialogue in an atmosphere of trust can add immeasurably to the effectiveness of any textbook and to the general learning experience. This book is not a complete encyclopedia of its subject matter, but it does offer selected information and hopefully may be a catalyst to stimulate some readers to continue the study of ethics.

In the area of personal mores, each individual has an image of himself in his mind. This personal image is projected to others through behavior patterns, mannerisms and style of dress and hair. It takes time and experience to sort these personal images, accept some, reject others and replace rejected images with new ones. This is part of the development of a personal philosophy of ethics that is requisite to attaining some degree of individual emotional security. This personal security is basic to emotional maturity and an understanding and acceptance of professional ethics. Personal, professional and Association Principles of Ethics are included in the discussion.

In the past, most dental hygienists have taken their professional lives seriously, but many of them have overlooked the fact that that very professionalism committed them to even broader objectives. Today's young professionals are more aware of this obligation, but, being inexperienced, they still need to be stimulated to channel their thinking in an ethical direction. The various responsibilities of the dental hygienist are presented and the multifaceted challenges of selected current issues are given consideration.

Even though the professional person is completely ethical there are legal hazards connected with the practice of dentistry and dental hygiene. The dental hygienist is solely liable for some acts and jointly liable for others. It is therefore necessary to understand the nature of the law as it applies to the practice of dental hygiene. It is also necessary to be able to identify the illegal practice of dentistry, malpractice and negligent conduct. Some of the basic principles in the section on jurisprudence relate more specifically to dentistry, but dental hygienists need to be aware of the possibilities of legal entanglements of the dentist as well as of themselves so that they may help avoid office and personal problems.

The development of oral hygiene and dentistry has been recorded by a number of historians. One chapter in this book can present only the highlights of these chronicles. There are two notable changes in the History of Oral Hygiene. One change is sad in a sense, but exciting because it is a new discovery. We have assumed that Irene Newman was the first dental hygienist and that Dr. Fones established the first course in dental hygiene. Since no other schools or people were mentioned, and no one presented contradictory evidence, we adopted the implication as fact. Norma Albertal, doing research, found a statement in a book on dental practice management and wrote asking for clarification. The question sparked further research which produced evidence through Mildred Gilsdorf, a past president of ADHA, that a formal course for dental nurses and assistants was given in the Ohio College of Dental Surgery prior to Dr. Fones' course in Bridgeport, Connecticut.

Although students were not called dental hygienists the course offered dental hygiene subjects, basic sciences and dental assisting, both didactic and clinical. Bulletins of the Ohio College of Dental Surgery list the course beginning in 1910 through 1914. At that time it appears to have been discontinued, probably because of the strong and bitter opposition of Ohio dentists.

Additional facts from Ohio dentists who were in school at that time tell us that Dr. C. M. Wright taught his dental assistant to perform dental hygiene procedures. No year is given, nor do we know her name, but it is possible that she was trained earlier than Mrs. Newman. However, as Miss Gilsdorf, the first licensed dental hygienist in Ohio, says. "Being first isn't all that important, as I can well testify. It's just what you do with being first that counts—when the standard is thrust in your hand you know you must accept the responsibility of leadership." Records of early dental hygienists as well as those of the American Dental Hygienists' Association were carefully researched in order to provide a comprehensive history of the Association. Many details had to be omitted, but the growth and development of significant Association programs are included. Chronology tables offer a capsuled but fairly complete history of the evolution of oral hygiene and the Association. Another chart gives an overview of constituent association formation, first legal practice of the dental hygienist, date of establishment and number of schools and the number of practicing dental hygienists in each state.

This book did not develop overnight. It is the result of years of thought, days and weeks of research, and lectures to and feed-back from students. It is not finished, it cannot be, for life is not static and ethics and ethical challenges must continually be practiced to be useful.

Books are seldom the product of individual effort. Many persons are involved through offering encouragement, support and understanding as well as active participation. Mrs. Patricia Wagner, Mrs. Irene Navarre, dental hygienists, and Mr. Daniel B. Keeling, attorney, and lecturer in Jurisprudence at the School of Dentistry, University of Southern California, reviewed and constructively criticized the first edition of this book. Additions and changes are in response to reader comments received and updated facts.

Robert H. W. Strang, M.D., D.D.S., an instructor of the first Fones' class of dental hygienists, and Miss Mabel McCarthy, an early Fones' graduate and a past president of the Association, now deceased, contributed to the history of dental hygiene. Anita Junck and Mrs. Elizabeth Entriken Barney, early California dental hygienists who were instrumental in the formation of the American Dental Hygienists' Association, also assisted with extensive historical information.

Northridge, California   WILMA E. MOTLEY

Contents

Chapter 1

Philosophy of Ethics

Overview of Ethics

"Ethics," a moral concept, has been considered worthy of major contemplation almost from the beginning of human life on earth. The notions of ethics in the beginning were very primitive, but the first unconscious glimmerings were there. Adam and Eve sensed intuitively that there was a right and a wrong way of doing things and they also quickly found that there were rewards and punishments connected with their actions. They soon learned that if they had privileges there were also concomitant duties and obligations. Before long they became concerned with such things, perhaps as yet unnamed, as justice, loyalty and honor. The thousands of years that passed were filled with growth in mental abilities and modifications in attitudes.

The original ethical concept was based upon mysticism. Tracing the history of ethics, we find it progressing gradually into the world of mystery which speculates on the unknown. Then, when man began to accumulate and record knowledge, he based his concepts on facts.

Man's interest in his destiny and belief in life hereafter are found first in the history of Egypt then in that of Babylonia. The belief that life here influenced life hereafter was evidenced in these philosophic writings and codes of conduct. *The Egyptian Book of the Dead,* dated 3500 B.C., describes immortality of the soul and lists behavior conducive to a desirable destiny.

Prior to 1000 B.C., India produced the *Vedas* which is the ancient, sacred literature of their society. Among expanded versions of the *Vedas* are the first philosophic writings, the *Upanishads,* remarkable for their discourses on many problems such as ethics, God, death and immortality. It was not until approximately 470 B.C. that Greek philosophy evolved. Representative among the early philosophers are Aristotle, whose realistic theories were based on facts within his experience, and Plato, who was idealistic and expounded on principles. According to these Greek philosophers, one's action was either right or wrong, based entirely on the philosophy of the individual's group.

Perhaps in early Greek civilization it was possible to have a code of ethics and follow it with little or no deviation. Because their way of living was less sophisticated and because they were not faced with the multiplicity of situations which confront the Twentieth Century civilization, it was reasonable for them to hold one philosophy or to accept one belief in its entirety. Living in today's realistic world, modern man finds it difficult, if not impossible, to apply idealistic ethics to everyday situations without many compromises. Only by accepting parts of philosophic theories and harmonizing them can he form realistic, functional ethical principles.

Compromise is a device used when one is willing to reject a part of his belief and substitute a part of that of another, so the change is made only when an agreement is more desirable. All people of any age daily use compromise as a tool to attain their goals or to retain what they have already achieved. A committee or commission report seldom reflects the complete wish or will of any member of the group, but it is a compromise which all members accept because it is an adjustment which enables continued action and progress. A function of government is to arrange compromise between conflicting group interests.

When interests are evenly balanced, two courses of action may be available. If both actions could solve the problem, then relative values of proceeding in either manner need to be judged in order to reach a decision. The action which leads to the most acceptable consequences or the action of greatest moral value should be the one chosen.

Throughout periods when European civilization developed, the process of evolution influenced the philosophy of ethics. The good man was the good citizen, a member of the hereditary elite who governed the Greek city-state. There was no science as it is now recognized and, without science there was no technology. For the Greeks, all philosophy was directed toward the activities of the elite because they had leisure time, and discussing philosophy was a way of using their free time. They were deeply concerned with man and his world and encouraged each other, particularly the young men, to develop an interest in nature and in the real man. The qualities of mind, intelligence, knowledge, action and the pursuit of truth, were valued highly and were considered virtues.

During the Middle Ages, philosophy and religion, united by a common ethical interest, transferred old theories to a new setting. Attitudes changed from considering what men ought to attempt to what they actually attempted. The importance of the individual as emphasized by Christianity became more widely accepted and scientific discoveries sparked the revival of learning. The Church did not encourage moral speculation; instead, it maintained that the Bible encompassed all standards of right and wrong. Scholars, refusing to accept this dogma, sought other standards of moral judgment.

The early modern period was more naturalistic and less religious; it was a compromise between the classical period and the Middle Ages. With the rise of science it was reasonable that man would try to measure everything by given standards, thus changing his approach to ethics and philosophy. This became a time of free will, and the nature and use of free will became an ethical issue. What ought to be and what was were topics for oral debate and written essay. The increasing democratization of society and the industrial revolution influenced changes in ethical philosophy as the value of the individual and his political responsibility underwent upheaval. As society became more complex it demanded changes and diversity of thought to fit its new sophistication.

The Nineteenth Century was, generally, a time of equality and plenty for all. While equality and plenty were not universally shared, they were possible for the first time. Although precise evidence cannot be found for correct conduct, the scientific theory became more pronounced during these years.

The Twentieth Century brought a great variety of moral beliefs, allowing a freedom in which each man could select his own values. The kinds of values selected depend on the individual's background, previous experiences, and ability or desire to be open-minded. Although technology makes it possible for man to do almost anything, science cannot answer man's moral dilemmas because it cannot distinguish between right and wrong and cannot insure against abuses. Although scientific methods can be used to evaluate ethical beliefs, scientific findings cannot induce man to pursue a better way of conduct unless he desires or is able to utilize services to this effect.

Philosophies of Ethics

Era	Approach	Representative	Belief
3500 B.C.	Egypt, Babylonia: Life now influenced hereafter	Egyptian Book of the Dead	Conduct, immortality were important
1000 B.C.	India: ethics, God, immortality	Vedas, Upanishads	God, death, immortality

470 B.C.	Greek: classical; idealism in ethics, one code for all	Socrates, Plato, Aristotle	Man should attempt to achieve perfection
Middle Ages	Philosophy and religion guided conduct	Thomas Aquinas	Happiness through love of God
		Niccolo Machiavelli	State as center of moral life
Early Modern	Less religious, more naturalistic society; became more democratic; time of free will	John Locke	Justified Christian religion as fundamentally reasonable
		Baruch Spinoza	To live according to reason is highest good
Eighteenth Century	Period of enlightenment; comparative religion debated; analyses of man's being and place in nature	Joseph Butler	Basis of morality is conscience
		Immanuel Kant	Duty not pleasure is highest conduct
		Jeremy Bentham	Moral value based on consequences
Nineteenth Century	Independent theories; modernistic tendencies; scientific methods;	John Stuart Mill	Ends, not means, are important, man should seek pleasure
		Herbert Spencer	Evolution of ethics
		Henry Sidgwick	Universal moral principles
		Thomas H. Green	Self-realization
Twentieth Century	Social philosophy; scientific method; religious aspects; all major aspects of philosophy	Hastings Rashdall	Applied ethical theory to practical life
		George E. Moore	Intuition
		John Dewey	Life is movement

Nature of Ethics

From time immemorial, philosophers have discussed and written about ethics. But, what is ethics? Ethics is the philosophy of human conduct, a way of stating and evaluating principles by which problems of behavior can be solved. Psychology, sociology and anthropology also are concerned with human conduct, but in different ways. Their function is to describe how and why men act as they do. Ethics is not concerned with description and explanation, but with evaluation of human conduct and with standards for judging whether actions are right or wrong.

Is ethics a science? The answer depends largely upon the definition of science. If the term "science" is used in a broad sense, meaning "any body of facts in a particular sphere classified and systematized" then ethics is a science. To know what exists is a natural science; to know what should matter is ethics. The fact that ethics is concerned with the ends, ideals or values involved in certain forms of activity distinguishes it from the natural sciences. It is the science of what is morally right. The interest is in discovering what ought to be right, not merely in discovering what is right. Ethics attempts to determine the goal or goals of living and to show men the means of attaining these goals. Knowledge of a science such as ethics is not "scientific" until it is accepted by those who know, such as those who have spent time in reflective philosophy and whose theories have been tested and accepted by many authorities. Ethical scientists and philosophers aim at as complete a knowledge of their subject as possible and constantly search for and find new facts.

Descriptions of the modern sciences are limited to one set of facts or objects, describing what man's sense organs tell him. Scientific descriptions do not involve value judgment. Psychologists study the mental processes leading to conduct without concern for whether or not the conduct is good or bad. Conduct is studied by sociologists who consider the institutions and customs of society which form the basis for individual behavior within that society. Anthropologists study conduct; although the entire human race is properly within their sphere of research, they have concerned themselves mainly with the characteristics of primitive man.

Another group of sciences, the normative sciences of aesthetics, logic and ethics, deals with how man makes judgments. Aesthetics, dealing with the doctrines of tastefulness, concerns the standards of perception. Logic, the art of exact reasoning, concerns the standards necessary to judge the validity or falsity of statements. Ethics evaluates conduct and judges actions to be right or wrong. Normative sciences go beyond the description of standards of judgment and, in addition, provide evidence of the validity of those standards and reasons for following them.

Sociology somewhat parallels ethics in its study and description of standards at different times and places. The sociologist may say that under certain circumstances polygamy is right for Mohammedans but that Christians reject it in favor of monogamy. This is a statement of fact and is not a value judgment which would state that one belief is right and the other wrong. Ethics states which actions one should believe and follow and provides standards by which right and wrong, good and bad can be judged. Ethics can study actions and assist one in analyzing and explaining his ethical judgments.

The word "moral" comes from the Latin *mos-mores* which means custom or way of life. The related word "ethics" is derived from the Greek word *ethos* meaning custom or character. Both terms refer to that type of behavior which tends to become customary because of the approval or practices of the group; thus, they are essentially synonymous. However, the words "morals" and "morality" usually refer to the conduct or system or code which is followed. Ethics attempts to determine what conduct or what actions ought to be approved or disapproved. It undertakes to furnish standards which distinguish between a better character and a worse one.

Ethics is not an object, such as an orange or a box, which one can hold in his hand, nor can one reach out and touch it or even point to it as he points to a star or a mountain top. It is as nebulous as a sigh or a thought. It cannot be bought, sold or bartered, but it can be shared. Ethics, like gravity, is with man all the time, usually without any self-awareness, or consciousness, but sometimes he does sense its strong, magnetic attraction. When man is stimulated by this influence, he is inclined to gravitate toward the ethical pole which was established early in his life.

No one can deny that the thick, sturdy, pungent peel of an orange makes a neat and tidy container for the juicy segments of fruit within, preserving them until someone is ready to feast the eye and satiate the appetite. Like an orange, although it has no tangible outer covering, ethics can be divided into segments and it awaits for someone to reflect on its ramifications in order to promote its significance in life, both personal and professional. Unlike the orange, ethics cannot be consumed; ethics is everlasting and is never lost.

The housekeeper makes use of various sizes and types of boxes to safeguard valuable objects and store others. Like a box, ethics can be divided into compartments, each with its own treasure. Unlike a box, ethics has no specific dimensions but it is ever expanding in its concepts and applications.

Early navigators, such as the Vikings, followed centuries later by Columbus and other explorers, depended on stars to guide them across uncharted seas. The Bible describes the journey of the Three Wise Men across the desert. Like a star, ethics is a compass to guide one through the maze of situations presented by life. Even though stars may be obscured by bright sunshine in the daytime or by clouds at night, they are always in their appointed places in the universe, and so is ethics. David, the Biblical psalmist, said, "I will lift up mine eyes unto the hills from whence cometh my help." Ethics may be considered the hills of help for modern man for, the more he studies ethics and the more he uses ethical concepts as guides, the more he is strengthened in character.

Continued reading and reflection about ethics only prove how complex and complicated a science it is. A serious study of ethics necessitates approaching it as a multi-disciplined subject. One book or one course in ethics only opens the door to understanding the many viewpoints, the many subdivisions of its scope.

Development of Morality

Sometimes vaguely, many times imperfectly, but always in some manner, moral standards have been expressed by man. The formally educated philosopher does not make up his own rules, but collects and systematizes the available information and records it in an orderly unbiased fashion. The theorist does not start with abstract principles and then build a theory; he studies the common mores of his contemporaries, criticizes them and arranges them in a system which, necessarily, is influenced by existing conditions of the period and by the mores with which he began. Established and generally accepted standards of behavior are evaluated critically to reveal inconsistencies, and the means of removing these contradictions are studied. Then, and only then, hypotheses may be formed, weighed, modified, accepted or rejected as facts indicate. Acceptance by a majority of men may indicate that an hypothesis is correct but acceptance does not necessarily prove that it is always correct, for there are still times when insight or intuition play a part in making decisions.

The moralist or moralizer, commonly known as the homespun philosopher, untrained in formal methods, has gained his knowledge through experience. The morals upon which he relies are not products of his mind, as are those of the philosopher, but are criteria observed through a lifetime of experience. Much literature is moralistic since it is a way in which writers explore real situations and express their convictions. Because of this common-sense philosophic observation of people and events over many years, the moralist's insight often deserves respect and credence.

Whether or not man naturally is free and good, or whether man seeks only that which pleases him, is a point which can be left to philosophers, but the development of morality in the human race can be traced through three stages: instinct, custom and conscience. Although man has advanced in developing morality, all levels of society show traces of each stage.

At the level of instinct, man's behavior appears right to him and his actions are responses to his fundamental needs and stimuli. The first need of any organism is to live and grow, so its first impulses and activities are for food, self-defense and other immediate necessities. The life of lower animals, which is life at its most instinctive level, cannot compare favorably with that of human society although the two have some instincts in common. Instinctive actions of lower animals usually are not considered right or wrong since apparently there is no judgment involved as there may be in the actions of human beings. A mother cat instinctively fights to protect her young, as do humans, and wild animals instinctively kill smaller animals as a source of food for themselves and their young. It must be assumed that there is some obscure feeling of the act being right, and thus it must have appeared in the beginning to man. One can presume that primitive man regarded as "right" those things which he found pleasurable, and "wrong" or "bad" those things which displeased him.

The first unit of society was the family. At some time, through the natural instinct of socializing, man formed associations with other men. Through mutually beneficial associations in a family group came a typical division of labor and an interchange of services. The man, being stronger, was the hunter and protector of the home and family; the woman, because her duties involved being a mother, stayed at home and performed household functions in the cave. The mother, very young children, and the very old members of the clan remained at the base of operations, participating in the group's activities as their abilities allowed. The woman, accidentally dropping a piece of fresh meat in the fire and not wanting to waste it, discovered that it tasted good when it was partially burned and warmed, even more palatable than when it was cold and raw. She also discovered that it kept better, and, as a result, man did not have to hunt every day. When hunting was good, affording an oversupply of meat, someone wove grasses into the shape of a basket to provide storage facilities. Spears, bows and arrows, cooking and storage pots, and division of labor progressed naturally, each step forward being necessitated by growth of the clan and, in turn, accelerating the clan's growth. Eventually men more skilled in certain arts became craftsmen of various kinds, and an exchange of services and objects developed into trade between tribes. Conduct became more skilled as man learned to use his intelligence in reasoning, finding that smaller, less hostile man could win an argument through use of brain power rather than brawn.

At this point, certain actions become "customary." Customs actually practiced eventually become approved standards and modes of behavior. Those things which have not been done in the past automatically are considered "bad." Approved conduct and certain behaviors are handed down from generation to generation. The young are trained to follow an established pattern, elders believing that, since the group always does this and approves it, always has done and approved it, it is well to continue the pattern and dangerous to deviate. At the customary level it is the whole tribe or community which is involved in right or wrong behavior. If one person is a wrongdoer, all persons in the tribe suffer. Primitive tribes in parts of the world ranging over the south seas to Africa, to northern India, to the Americas have had, or still have, blood feuds in which a victim is avenged only by punishment of many or all of the wrongdoer's family.

Customs have always been ways of acting which appeased and contented the whole group, either fulfilling unsophisticated desires or representing a compromise of feelings within the group. Just because a catastrophe befalls the group the day someone happens to break a custom does not mean that catastrophe will always occur when the custom is violated. But at this level of intelligence it is believed so and the custom becomes a superstition. To the primitive man "tabu" indicated that there is a punishment for breaking some custom and he believed that supernatural forces, perhaps through a dead ancestor, would inflict dire punishment on the person who had performed the forbidden act. Because man has sought approval, religious ritual and public opinion have been, and still are, very powerful in enforcing customs and tabus. Much importance has been placed on ritual and it has been expressed in many ways: the ritual of administering the oath of office to the president of the United States, to presidents of organizations and to judges of our courts; rituals of the courts of law; rituals concerned with birth, marriage and death; the ritual of breaking ground for new construction or topping off a new building. The power of public opinion has been evidenced and documented in man's political and social lives.

Man finds it simple to follow customary morality because it has provided standards, relieving him of the necessity to rely on what he thinks is right or wrong or what appeals to him. Acceptance of customs, on the whole, is a social gain for there would be no stability in mores if everyone questioned custom, and young people would have no lasting guides for conduct. The outward observance of custom satisfies the group itself but the inflexible moral standard slows down progress since it does not allow flexibility for individual variation or growth. If customary moral standards are to be enforced strictly, they cannot be set very high. Instead they must be maintained at a level the average person is capable of achieving. Punishment for violating custom may keep the individual up to the level of morality but there is nothing in custom to urge him to achieve above-average morality.

In periods of customary morality one merely follows custom; it is in periods of reflective morality that real progress is made in man's moral evolution. When man begins to investigate within himself the causes of conduct, rather than outward actions, his moral life is enlarged and he finds that morality is something he can understand. It is only when man advances to the level of conscience that moral authority becomes an individual activity and man's actions can contradict group behavior, for his actions depend entirely on what he thinks is right. He may even speculate on the customs of the group, discovering that certain customs no longer may be useful, that they may even be deleterious, not fulfilling their original purposes, and that certain customs, such as slavery, cannot be justified by moral reflective thinking. Man has always looked for the new while clinging to the old, customary ways and beliefs. It is only when he discovers inconsistencies in thought or action that he is willing to consider change.

Conscience can give rise to a sense of uneasiness for it is a product of individual experience and social contacts. It is a name for the restraining impulses upon conduct which come from within the individual, the feeling of obligation to do or not to do certain things. It may be a vague reluctance arising out of unfamiliarity in the presence of the new or untried. It may be social pressure to conform or it may be the individual conviction that the action is harmful in its personal or social effects. Conscience is not infallible, for repeated wrong actions can dull its reactions and cause it to be quiescent, outside influences can modify it, or reflection and experience can cultivate and discipline it.

Theory of Ethics

There is a division of thought on the purpose of studying ethics: some believe it is a purely theoretical subject; others believe that its essential purpose is to change our actions. The majority maintain that it is primarily a theoretical study, seeking the truth about morality, but that, in studying the subject, ethics becomes a practical matter. No matter which philosophy one accepts, if one carefully studies various theories, one finds that these theories do not disagree to any great extent. The theorist is inclined to overlook practical applications of ethics and the practical student will overlook the theory of ethics. Theorists can outline untrue theories; the practical student can lose sight of broad principles involved. Our philosophy determines our ethical standards. Our personal moral beliefs develop as we associate with others. These beliefs can, and some will, change as they are influenced by another's viewpoint.

Because man lives in society with other people, not completely alone, he has many loyalties, some stronger than others. He is a part of the state, but also a part of the family, church, school, club and business, and he is an individual. In spite of the many affiliations and differing obligations imposed, man still is the unit of which these groups are composed and his actions are those with which ethics is concerned.

Man must often decide a course of action based on what is best at the moment, for too many times no available alternate choice is ideal. If ethical behavior is to mean the choice of the better of possible situations, and it often is, then ethics is a part of man's life almost from the day he is born. His first concept of morals is implanted by parents, later by companions and teachers. As a child his experiences are limited; as an adult he is still open to suggestion. Long before he is aware of it, he practices ethics in his daily living. The baby who learns to share the attention of parents with others is taking the first step in the direction of ethical behavior and, as he grows older, he learns not only to share affection but also material possessions with brothers, sisters and friends and to make minor ethical decisions.

There are two fundamental truths which our society believes every child should be taught: to mind his mother and to tell the truth. When he goes to a birthday party he is reminded by mother to thank his hostess and to tell her that he had a good time. At the party another guest teases and hits him and, as he finally leaves for home, he is faced with a decision. Is he going to mind his mother and tell his hostess he had a good time, which is obviously a lie, or is he going to be honest with his hostess, perhaps hurt her feelings, and certainly disobey his mother? While we might class this as a minor ethical decision it is of major importance the first time it is faced and may be the beginning of ethical awareness.

Systems of justice are based on whether or not a person could have made some other choice, and systems of rewards and punishments, praise and blame, approval and disapproval assume that there is freedom of choice and responsibility. People are held responsible for their acts according to their age and intelligence.

As a first step toward growth and improvement, man must learn to accept himself, his handicaps, and his limitations, as well as his abilities and achievements. Also, he must learn to accept other people and the world in which he lives. There are limitations which can be changed and man should work toward those changes which are good, or should work to modify or accept those things which cannot be changed. To know in which direction to move, man needs a faith, a set of consistent ideals, a philosophy of life, for he tends to become what he imagines he is. Socrates reportedly said, "The shortest and surest way to live with honor in the world is to be in reality what we would appear to be; all human virtues increase and strengthen themselves by the practice and experience of them."

When man no longer believes that the universe supports in some measure his highest aspirations and ideals he begins to lose heart and there seems to be a note of sadness and futility about his life. Religion or a firm philosophic belief gives meaning to his life, supplying the faith, the ideals and the philosophy he must develop in order to grow and improve. Common to all faiths, differing as they do, is the offer of hope for a better life and definite directions for its attainment by followers of that faith.

Moral Standards

There are many approaches to solving the complex problems presented by ethics but, first, principles of judgment to be used must be stated and evaluated. To know what is right is one ethical problem, yet to do what is right is another. Before we can determine which behavior is right or wrong, good or bad, there must be standards by which to judge the action. Conduct is action; action can be voluntary or involuntary. While some philosophers consider both types of actions, ethics is concerned primarily with voluntary actions, including motives and intentions as well as muscular movements and articulation. In other words, ethics is concerned with conduct which can consciously be controlled. Judgments of character and motives are important, but since these judgments depend finally on the judgment of observed behavior, it can be assumed that some knowledge of the basis for moral judgment of voluntary actions is an asset to the dental hygienist. Over the years many methods for evaluating moral standards have been proposed, and for each school of thought there have been arguments for and against, as well as proposals for modifications and adaptations of each of them. Among criteria offered are standards of judgment based on Intuition, Law, Pleasure, Evolution, Perfection and Value. A serious study of philosophy reveals that no school of thought and no standard of judgment stands as a law unto itself. Each one has overtones of at least one other, basing its rationale on a slightly different viewpoint. Circumstances seem to sway us toward one belief or another in order to adjust to our immediate environmental situation, all within proper ethical limitations.

Intuition, equated with conscience by Butler, is common to all people and is an automatic reaction, a result of past moral influences. Intuitionism, as defined by Moore in his *Principa Ethica,* regards the good as "indefinable" and confines its theory to the fact that the only criterion for judging actions right or wrong is by intuition, not reflection. The experienced person intuitively knows right action, just as the dental hygienist knows from habit, not reflection, which instrument to use in a given area of the mouth.

Sidgwick noted that we may intuitively believe that lying is always wrong, but if a lie would save a man's life, and we also believe that it is right to save human life, how can we say lying is wrong in this case? Is the soldier, captured by the enemy, justified in saying he has no information about his country's defenses, although he does have, in order to protect his country and countrymen?

Kant was one of many who believed that nature's laws, which are laws of reason, and the conservation, welfare or happiness of its beings, should be the criteria for evaluation of moral standards. These laws, he said, should be applicable to all people and that perfect harmony of the will with moral law is the ultimate goal, although admittedly it is a goal unattainable in life. It was Kant's belief that following duty, not pleasure, was the highest type of conduct for man.

Moral laws keep us from actions which are bad, but they cannot guide us to the complete fulfillment of human goodness. No law, civil, scientific or moral, can demand unique actions such as heroism often demonstrated in war or in stress situations, for it is the spirit in which an action is taken, or not taken, as much as the action itself which gives it moral value.

Mill, who associated pleasure with good, believed that man exists best with pleasure and without pain, and that the ends, not means, were important standards of judgment. Some philosophers declare that there are differences in the quality of pleasure, others argue that there are differences in the value of the pleasure engendered. Still others express the opinion that all pleasures are of equal quality and value.

Influenced by Darwin's theories, Spencer was one of the main proponents of the Evolutionary Theory as a standard for evaluation of moral judgment. He believed that better conduct is merely more evolved conduct, and he traced the evolution of conduct from animals to humans to society as he knew it. Since he believed that the physiologic life was inseparable from the psychologic life, then it followed that social evolution and moral standards paralleled biologic evolution. Society itself has evolved from a homogeneous structure of the family into the heterogeneous complex system of many families living together in many diverse groups with accompanying changes in moral conduct. To Spencer, "survival of the fittest" meant that good conduct was necessary for survival, and that the individual who survived practiced behavior beneficial to life, rising from what we call "good conduct" to "best conduct" as he achieved the ultimate in his life.

The theory of perfection in the judgment of moral standards is basically a spiritual one. Green's theory of absolute idealism was based on his belief that the mind within can be known only through reflection on itself which is centered on personal character rather than on the race. Perfectionists believe that goodness of conduct depends on the goodness of the result to which it leads.

Ethical judgments are often based on values. The quality of an action, or an object, can be real or implied, for "values" are general judgments of the individual, although a substantial number of types of experiences are valued in much the same way all over the world. Rashdall tried to arrange intrinsic goods a man should aim for into a system of values, placing virtue first. Aristotle held that the contemplative life of a philosopher was of the highest value, and others place communion with God at the top of the list.

It is perfectly possible that more than one action can be right at one time as well as the existing possibility that only one action can be right at a given time. When more than one action is "right," a value judgment must be made. It can be as right for one to choose a cup of coffee as for another to choose a cup of tea. Since there is no ethical choice involved in the choosing, either action is right. But if one is choosing for himself and a friend, and he knows the friend has a preference, then the choice becomes one of ethical values. Moore says that the value should designate more than just a pleasant, happy experience; value should denote worth. He further states that, if value exists, it appears in both particular and general modes as a color appears in its general basic shade and also in hues of that general shade. He believes that one of the most valuable attributes a person might have is his attitude toward others.

Value is a sense of what is or should be right and what is or should be wrong according to each person's individual perception or experience. It can be expressed as a feeling or it can be a thought or an opinion. Value is not directly observable but the characteristics of value can be observed.

Rights and Duties

Ethical philosophers reflect upon rights, duties and virtue, for these things are a part of the good life. Rebels and reformers alike have listed the "rights" of man. The Declaration of Independence states that there are certain fundamental rights of man, as does the Five Freedoms of Roosevelt and Churchill. Rights may be justifiable claims or moral rights. Justifiable claims may be enforced by law, such as those enacted for the protection of property. Intangible moral rights, such as the right to respect, are unenforceable and must be earned. To be truly justifiable, fundamental claims and moral rights must lead to the common good. Knowing when to assert one's rights and when to compromise are the most important qualities for man to possess or to cultivate. The following are the fundamental rights of man as listed by Mackenzie: (1) the right to life, (2) the right to freedom, (3) the right to hold property, (4) the right of contract, and (5) the right to education. All of these rights, however, are subject to some limitations and interruptions.

Duty is the obligation to fulfill a right. Some duties and obligations are common to all people, others are peculiar to the individual as a consequence of his special abilities or circumstances. It may be an obligation of the individual to satisfy a claim of another individual or the community in return for certain rights given him. Duty may also involve several other individuals and may entail a further obligation of the recipient. For instance, the right to an education involves the duty of the parent or society to provide an education and also the duty of the student to use the education received for the good of society. It would be difficult, if not impossible, to outline all duties for any right because varying circumstances would point out addition of some duties and omission of others.

There are also moral obligations which are accepted in a different sense. Sensitive people feel that it is their duty to do certain things although there is no right to be gained, such as the urge to finish what one starts and the sense of obligation to some person or cause.

"Virtue," according to the Greek, means excellence. The four cardinal virtues described by Plato in his *Republic* are Wisdom, Courage, Temperance and Justice, to which medieval philosophers added the theological virtues of Faith, Hope and Love. A careful study of the discourses of Socrates and his peers yields insight into early thought on the good life as each of the virtues was fully discussed in a rational manner.

Virtue is a quality of character and may, by common usage, also be a practice which corresponds to that quality. A man's duty may be done through enforcement of law, with no agreeable feeling or willingness on his part, but if he voluntarily, with good will, goes farther than required, then his action is known as a virtue. Ethical theory makes no clear distinction between duty and virtue for they are matters of conscience, and conscience points out more duties to some men than to others. Those with lesser conscience then consider performance beyond their conscience of duty a virtue.

Summary

There is every reason to believe that, quite properly, there will be continued change in man's beliefs, for change indicates that philosophy and

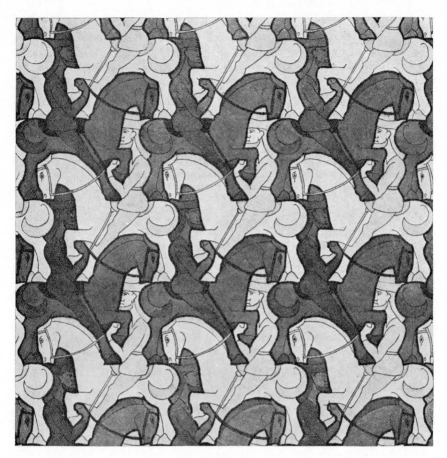

One of Maurits Escher's mathematical mosaics. (From Macgillavry, C. H.: *Symmetry Aspects of M. C. Escher's Periodic Drawings.* A. Oosthoek's Uitgeversmaatschappij N. V., Utrecht, 1965.)

ethics are living entities and concepts are constantly readapting to actual human situations while retaining the cardinal and theological virtues of Wisdom, Courage, Temperance, Justice, Faith, Hope and Love as basic guides.

Perhaps perfection in ethics cannot be attained, but it is a goal worthy to seek. Humans are not perfect, but constant striving for perfection is humanly possible. The more man tries to attain a degree of perfection, and the more he is guided by ethics, the easier it becomes for him to make appropriate decisions and to act wisely. Being ethical should become such a conscious habit that only occasionally will values need serious reflection.

Are ethics black or white? Is there a gray area? The picture above is for all to see, but not everyone sees the same thing. Some people first see the black knights on black horses, some will first see white knights on white horses. Most people will be able to see both the black and white knights and horses, but a few will see only one set of knights and horses. Can ethics be like this, with not everyone seeing the same values in a specific situation? Yes, for cultures and customs vary and influence the moral side of ethics, and there is much overlapping of philosophical, ethical theories. The final resolution of each circumstance is accomplished by the judgment of the individual whose decision is based on his background, his experience, his knowledge and the times in which he lives.

References

Avey, Albert E.: *Handbook in the History of Philosophy,* 2nd ed. New York, Barnes & Noble, 1962.

Jones, William T. et al.: *Approaches to Ethics,* 2nd ed. New York, McGraw-Hill Book Company, 1962.

Lillie, William: *An Introduction to Ethics,* 3rd ed. New York, Barnes & Noble, 1961.

Mackenzie, John S.: *Manual of Ethics,* 6th ed. London, University Tutorial Press Ltd., 1929.

Runes, Dagobert D.: *Dictionary of Philosophy.* Totowa, New Jersey, Littlefield Adams, 1965.

Chapter 2

Ethics of the Dental Hygienist

In order to have an orderly social organization, there must be agreements, understandings, principles or rules of procedure. Any cooperative group activity is founded upon conventions, customs and agreements which may be conscious and overtly evident or unconsciously embedded in the habits of its members. Ethics seeks the most intelligent principles of behavior, or the principles which will make life most wholesome.

In the moral development of the human race, guides and checks for conduct have developed. These guides and checks have been expressed outwardly in conventions, customs, legal and ecclesiastical laws, and in rules and codes of various kinds. They have been expressed inwardly in the sense of duty or the conscience of the individual, in shame and remorse, in praise and blame, or in contentment and dissatisfaction.

Man lives in a world in which he must not only make decisions but must also learn the right ways and wrong ways of doing things. He may possess great technical skill in business or in a profession yet be very stupid concerning his sense of values. No one can live a satisfactory life without having some scale of values. Ethics seeks to establish the true values of life.

Man's first need is to live and grow. His first impulses and activities are for nourishment, protection and other immediate necessities. When these needs are fulfilled, then the socializing side of the process of development begins, and the individual enters into relationships with other human beings. Eventually, cooperation, interchange of services and participation in associations evolve.

As families expanded, they developed into clans with customs and rituals. Certain ways of acting which were common to the group then became folk-ways. Approved actions were handed down from generation to generation, thus becoming part of the customs of the group. The young were carefully trained to perform these actions, for an act so sanctioned gains cumulative pressure.

Each class or group tends to develop its own mores or standards from which grow institutions and laws. Each group believes that its mores are good and that the standards of right and wrong are inherent in them. Be-havior ordinarily conforms to standards approved by groups trusted and admired, and individual moral ideals tend to sanction these ways. While there is very little that has not at some time or place been regarded as wrong, there is also very little that has not been approved by some group at some time. Thus, it becomes a fact that custom can make almost any-thing appear right or wrong. Man is inclined to go along with the crowd because he feels the moral sanction of group response.

A profession consists of a limited group of persons who have acquired some special skill and are therefore able to perform that function in society better than the average person. Alternatively stated, a profession is a calling the members of which profess to have acquired special knowledge by training or experience, or both, so that they may advise or serve others in that special field.

Certain characteristics are included in the general idea of a profession: (1) special preparation or training, (2) a clearly defined and comparatively permanent membership, and (3) the acceptance of the service motive. The professional person is expected to have respect for human beings, competence in his chosen field, integrity, and a primary concern with ser-vice rather than with prestige or profit.

Professional ethics, as distinct from morals and from law, gives atten-tion to certain additional ideals and practices which develop from an indi-vidual's professional privileges and responsibilities. Professional ethics, which applies to certain functional groups, is the expression of the attempt to define situations for that particular group, situations which would other-wise remain indefinite or uncertain. Ethical codes are the result of an attempt to direct the moral consciousness of the members of the profession to its peculiar problems. They crystallize moral opinion and define be-havior in these specialized fields.

In business the definite aim is the financial return; the professional ideal includes an acceptance of the "service" motive. Even though he does not always live up to the ideal, the professional person is expected to render his best service at all times in order to advance the public interest, quite apart from the amount of the reward. While the professional man usually depends upon fees or a salary, such considerations, ideally at least, should not be uppermost in his mind and the quality of the service rendered should not be dependent on the fee which is expected.

Specialization brings benefits but may also lead to development of "blind spots." The specialist may see life in segments or fragments. He may give his undivided attention to the technical side of his field and bestow little or no thought to the aspect of morals and the application of his special knowledge to human welfare. The more specialized the knowledge, the higher the skill, and the less the public knows about the quality and the technical aspects of the work, the greater the opportunity for abuses to arise. Consequently, there is a social need for codes and laws.

Medical and dental professions have set up definite standards to which individual members of the group must conform or lose their professional standing. Codes of ethics are important means of social control for they define professional conduct for the new member and help to keep the old member in line. Often the professional code of ethics prevents control or interference by the government or by society through some other agency. Ethical codes are important in developing higher standards of conduct, for they are based upon what is considered to be the correct attitude and the correct procedure. The codes crystallize what is usually the best opinion and judgment of the profession; thus, they tend to eliminate misunderstandings and conflicts. They enable the group to bring pressure to bear upon those who would lower the standing of the group or cast reflection upon its good name. Some codes are general statements of purposes and ideals, others contain definite sets of rules of conduct.

Development of Codes of Ethics

Every group, from the family to world government, has rules and regulations. These can be written, unwritten, or implied. The more complex the group, the more necessary are the details of these rules and regulations. Formally organized groups operate under guides known as constitutions and bylaws which are broad statements of duties and responsibilities, plus operational manuals which go into greater detail of functions of officers and committees. Constitutions and bylaws as well as articles of incorporation are formal documents changed only under specified circumstances, approved by a stated majority of voting members. Policies are voted upon by a House of Delegates or another authorized body, and definitive statements are based on these policies. Along with these documents are behavioral codes known as principles of ethics.

The first code was written by Hammurabi, a Babylonian king, in 2300 B.C. This code was actually the law of the land and exacted an "eye for an eye," a "tooth for a tooth," a law of retaliation.

Hippocrates is given credit for writing the first voluntary code of regulations for the medical profession, protecting the right of patients and appealing to the finer instincts of the physician. Sir Thomas Percival of England wrote a medical code in 1792, and in 1832 the American Medical Association based its first code on his writings. John Allen wrote the first code of ethics which was formally adopted by the American Dental Association in 1866.

Since 1890, hundreds of business and professional groups in the United States have adopted codes of ethics. Some of these codes which are more or less perfunctory are not taken very seriously by the membership. Nevertheless, the very fact of their being formulated exerts a pressure in the direction of higher standards.

The dental hygienist is relatively free of evaluation and control by laymen. The American Dental Hygienists' Association, while exercising absolute minimum control, constantly seeks to initiate higher standards imperative in these days of specialization, and has established guidelines for relations between members of the profession, dentistry and patients.

In 1926, during the third annual session of the American Dental Hygienists' Association, the first code of ethics for dental hygienists was adopted. Written in simple but clear phrases, it outlined the ethical responsibilities of members of the profession.

The Duties of the Profession to Their Patients

Section 1. The dental hygienist should be ever ready to respond to the wants of her patrons, and should fully recognize the obligations involved in the discharge of her duties toward them. As she is in most cases unable to correctly estimate the character of her operations, her own sense of right must guarantee faithfulness in their performance. Her manner should be firm yet kind and sympathizing so as to gain the respect and confidence of her patients, and even the simplest case committed to her care should receive that attention which is due to operations performed on living, sensitive tissue.

Section 2. It is not to be expected that the patient will possess a very extended or very accurate knowledge of professional matters. The dental hygienist should make due allowance for this, patiently explaining many things which seem quite clear to herself, thus endeavoring to educate the public mind so that it will properly appreciate the beneficent efforts of our profession. She should encourage no false hopes by promising success when in the nature of the case there is uncertainty.

Section 3. The dental hygienist should be temperate in all things, keeping both mind and body in the best possible health, that her patients may have the benefit of the clearness of judgment and skill which is their right.

From time to time the form and wording have been changed, but the basic guiding principles have not been altered.

For many years a detailed code of admonitions and prohibitions was in effect, but the House of Delegates of 1969 adopted more permissive statements of ethical behavior. An attempt was made to outline the ideals of the profession in broad statements.

Code of Professional Ethics for the Dental Hygienist

The philosophical, practical science of ethics establishes by reason and intelligent observation principles to direct our human conduct. Professional conduct incorporates the knowledge of these principles into practice. The following principles adopted by the 1974 House of Delegates constitute a guide to the responsibilities of the dental hygienist.

Each member of the American Dental Hygienists' Association has the ethical obligation to subscribe to the following principles:
To provide oral health care utilizing highest professional knowledge, judgment, and ability
To serve all patients without discrimination.
To hold professional patient relationships in confidence.
To utilize every opportunity to increase public understanding of oral health practices.
To generate public confidence in members of the dental health professions.
To cooperate with all health professions in meeting the health needs of the public.
To recognize and uphold the laws and regulations governing this profession.
To participate responsibly in this professional Association and uphold its purpose.
To maintain professional competence through continuing education.
To exchange professional knowledge with other health professions.
To represent dental hygiene with high standards of personal conduct.

Interpretation of ADHA Principles of Ethics

To provide oral health care utilizing highest professional knowledge, judgment and ability.

The dental hygienist within the limits of education and experience is constantly making decisions on care, treatment and education of the individual patient. Responsibility for these decisions must be accepted. The choice of an instrument and its use, the home care recommended, nutritional counseling are everyday examples of functions for which skilled judgment is required and for which responsibility must be assumed.

The dental hygienist must have the ability to recognize all abnormalities of the oral cavity and its supporting structures. These deviations from the normal must be brought to the attention of the dentist for his diagnosis and treatment. It then becomes the responsibility of the dentist to treat the pathology or refer the patient to the care of someone qualified in the particular specialty.

The dental hygienist is entitled to fair remuneration for the services performed in the dental office (or other place of employment) but this must be a fair exchange: competent care for patients and cooperation within the office structure in exchange for financial reimbursement. There can be no diminishment of proper procedures, no "short changing" in any manner. Each patient must be given the benefit of the best care the dental hygienist is capable of providing. The dentist must have the complete confidence of the dental hygienist and the staff must be treated fairly in a spirit of oneness.

The preventive, educational, and therapeutic procedures legally performed by the dental hygienist are being reevaluated in many states and procedures have already been extended in some. Through dental hygiene constituent associations and the national association, members have expressed their opinions which were transmitted as a consensus to dental associations and appropriate legal bodies.

To serve all patients without discrimination.

Discrimination can be based on the usually listed characteristics of race, creed, color, age, sex or cultural heritage, but it could also include physical or mental handicaps, financial status, occupation or appearance. Another form of discrimination is unwillingness to donate time to help care for those who need oral health services. Remuneration should not be the fundamental goal of the dental hygienist.

Regardless of any of these factors the human being who seeks or needs the care a dental hygienist can offer deserves consideration. Within established office policies the dental hygienist must be prepared to fulfill the professional obligation which was willingly accepted. It is not always easy but the majority of the time it proves to be an unexpectedly rewarding experience.

Students often have the opportunity to work with disadvantaged groups in inner city or rural areas as well as in hospitals and rehabilitation centers. Devices for aiding the handicapped in personal oral health maintenance have been fabricated by inventive dental hygienists and students.

To hold professional patient relationships in confidence.

This is not only an ethical precept but it is a legal requirement. The professional who discloses confidential information about one patient to another violates a trust and becomes potentially liable to be sued for slander. The patient who is told these facts will probably realize that his confidences may also be betrayed and his faith is destroyed. To hold professional patient relationships in confidence is a sure way of building and continuing professional and public esteem for the individual and the profession.

To utilize every opportunity to increase public understanding of oral health practices.

It would seem to be obvious that the dental hygienist would uphold the laws of the community; to understand them could be more difficult. In order to vote intelligently, it is necessary to study reasons for proposals to adopt or reject new laws or to modify existing laws. If the dental hygienist believes it advisable to participate actively in a campaign to adopt, reject or modify a law, then thorough study of and sincere belief in the cause are real necessities.

Dental hygienists should not wait to be asked to participate in community programs; they should initiate programs. The dental hygienist often works with the dental society in promoting National Children's Dental Health Week programs, community fluoridation projects and career day presentations. Other opportunities could be promoted and it should not be difficult to initiate joint projects with dental assistants, women's auxiliary groups, nurses, teachers or other health-oriented groups. Many dental hygiene societies have sponsored philanthropic projects which give dental care and education to children, handicapped persons or geriatric patients.

The former ADHA Principles of Ethics state "A dental hygienist may properly participate in a program of health education of the public involving such media as the press, radio, television, and lectures, providing that such programs are in keeping with the dignity of the profession and the custom of the dental profession of the community." Although this is no longer written policy it is still a precept to be followed. It is advisable to seek approval of the component or constituent association before participating in such programs. These endeavors must not advertise the services of the specific dental hygienist nor should office addresses or telephone numbers be used.

To generate public confidence in members of the dental health professions.

Disruption of the harmony which should exist among the members of the office staff may be a result of an unfounded sense of importance engendered by the unbalanced ratio of dental hygienists to dentists and dental assistants and to the acquisition of licensure. Each member of the dental health team has an important role, and the effectiveness of the team is lost when one individual assumes an undeserved importance. As a reasonable human being, the dental hygienist should make every effort to adjust to others and work cooperatively with them. The dental hygienist is not obligated to have confidence in the other members of the dental team, but, if it is not possible to function harmoniously with them or have confidence in them, employment should be sought elsewhere. Some constituent Principles of Ethics state that it is unethical for a dental hygienist to continue employment with a dentist who offers sub-standard services to patients.

Former Principles of Ethics state that "The dental hygienist thas the obligation of not referring disparagingly to the services of another dental hygienist or dentist in the presence of a patient. A lack of knowledge of conditions under which the services are afforded may lead to unjust criticism and to a lessening of the patient's confidence in the dental profession." Students question this principle. Is the dental hygienist to protect an inferior practitioner and let the patient suffer from improper care? Because patients often do not report their complaints accurately, it should first be determined whether the lack of care was due to the practitioner's incapability or to the reluctance or uncooperativeness of the patient. Will telling the patient honestly that the dental care has been substandard lessen his confidence in the dental profession? Is the greater responsibility to the profession or to the patient? The choices must be weighed carefully and the decision made with each individual case.

To cooperate with all health professions in meeting the health needs of the public.

Dental hygienists have always worked with other dental health professional groups but it could be easy to overlook additional opportunities for community service. Medicine, nursing, therapy, and even legislative agencies should be included among these related professions. A growing awareness of total needs of all people has increased the participation of dental hygiene in community, state and national activities.

Activities which help meet the health needs of the public are not confined to actual clinical services but include planning and/or supervising health care programs; acting as consultant to developing programs; actively supporting legislation which affects health and health care.

To recognize and uphold the laws and regulations governing this profession.

One hundred years ago the practice of dentistry was entirely up to the individual. It was after dentists worked together as an association that dental schools were established and licensing regulated. The practice of dentistry today is changing from solo practice to group practice, and the responsibility of the patient to pay for his care is also changing from individual responsibility to insurance plans of some type. Federal government insurance is the next step. The practice of dental hygiene is also in transition.

The dental hygienist follows the laws of the state, practicing under the supervision of a licensed dentist. Preferably the dentist is a member of a recognized dental association, certainly one who practices in a comparable ethical manner, showing concern for the patient's welfare.

The dental hygienist performs only those procedures allowed by the laws of the place of practice. Even though extended functions have been taught in school, or are allowed by some jurisdictions, the dental hygienist is to follow the rules and regulations of the area of practice. Students have suggested that in following this principle another is being violated. They are taught that service rendered the patient is to be optimum, consistent with the dental hygienist's training and education, and that the needs of the patient are the prime concern of the professional office. Must the dental hygienist withhold from the patient some portion of oral health care to which he is entitled, and which is a formally learned skill, as a consequence of differing laws?

Many changes in federal and state laws which affect the practice of dental hygiene are being proposed. Only through the representative voice of an association can effective action be taken. Legislation includes the expanding Association programs. All proposals are studied and then recommendations are made. Only statements that conform to Association policies are used. Every dental hygienist, practicing or nonpracticing, regardless of age, should be interested in these legalities and should find it vital to future professional health to belong to the Association. Through the Association, the dental hygienist is able to make opinions known. How else can this profession be protected and upgraded for future generations?

The terms "unethical" and "illegal" may often be confused. Unethical practices should be reported to the local professional society for review and counselling. Illegal practices are reported to the state board of dental examiners for their investigation and action. The dental hygienist should be very sure of facts and willing to support them before taking such action.

The Advisory Opinions of the Principles of Ethics of the American Dental Association state that it is unethical for a dentist to include the name of a dental hygienist on his cards, letterheads or office door. (Sec. 13, Advisory Opinion 9; Section 14, Advisory Opinion 3, Jan. 1, 1973.) The interpretation is that the dentist who allows this is unethical because he is thus advertising that he offers a service not all dentists can offer.

Many dental hygienists do not understand why names on cards, letterheads or doors are so important to ethics, for their concept of ethics is that it is a "people matter," an appropriate functioning of human relationships.

To participate responsibly in this professional Association and uphold its purpose.

When administrators and instructors in dental hygiene programs are interested in the Association and promote it, the example of their own active participation motivates the student to join the professional organization and become an active member in fact as well as in name. Changes in the ADHA Bylaws which give student members more privileges should encourage application for and use of full membership. National membership for a year after graduation is being considered. Junior members are included on some committees and their use as consultants on other committees will promote more interest and more awareness. Better communications between active and student members are necessary for it is a fact that members who are not aware of organizational activities cannot be expected to be interested. It is also suggested that constituent and component dental hygiene organizations make bylaw changes which would give junior members corresponding privileges in these groups.

"There is a time and place for everything" is an old adage. The time for membership in the dental hygiene association is now and always, for all dental hygienists. Only by representing a majority of the profession can the association be an authentic voice for dental hygiene.

The time and place for activity in the dental hygiene organization may vary as family responsibilities change. Component participation should be encouraged and with experience more responsibility can be accepted at constituent and national levels. Full participation will provide a continually expanding, satisfying experience.

If Association programs are to be instituted and existing programs offering more service to members are to be expanded, the need for financial support increases. It is vital to the profession that as services grow, so must membership support.

The economic status of the dental hygienist in civil service or the armed forces is determined by the ratings of those agencies. From time to time the Association has aided in upgrading these ratings and will continue to do so as indicated.

The economic status of the dental hygienist in private practice is determined by agreement between the dental hygienist and the employing dentist. The responsibility should remain with these two involved professionals. To give the responsibility for this determination to a third party would reduce dental hygiene to a vocation or trade, thus destroying its professional status.

The objectives, or purposes, of the Association have not changed appreciably over the years although their wording has become more altruistic in keeping with today's aims of health professionals. The latest revision, which will not be voted on until the 1975 annual meeting states: "The purposes of the Association are to improve the oral health of the public, to advance the art and science of dental hygiene, to maintain the highest standards of dental hygiene education and practice, to represent and protect the interests of the dental hygiene profession, to improve the professional competence of the dental hygienist, to foster research in oral health, and to provide professional communications; all in a manner consistent with the Principles of Ethics of the profession."

To maintain professional competence through continuing education.

Professional skills and judgment are improved through continual use. Constant advances in scientific knowledge and techniques make it necessary to add knowledge and skills to those originally learned. In order to give the patient the quality of care to which he is entitled, the dental hygienist must continue education throughout professional life. Books, professional journals, lectures and discussion groups add to this fund of knowledge but do not replace formal postgraduate study in an educational institution. These courses can vary from an evening to a full year of study. Some states are already requiring evidence of continuing education for licensure renewal and others are considering such legal action. It seems regrettable that the law must prescribe what an ethical concept should have motivated.

If research were not conducted there would be no scientific advancement and few empirical alterations of practice. Not every dental hygienist has the education, aptitude or facilities to conduct scientific research but each has an obligation to help further the work of others. Recorded observations by a number of dental hygienists could stimulate research projects or aid in verifying research statistics.

To exchange professional knowledge with other health professions.

For many years dentistry has believed that new discoveries which further the health care of the public should be shared. An exchange of professional knowledge with other health professions would include such activities as: routinely reading other professional publications; writing articles for other publications, and accepting theirs; attending or giving lectures to other professions; attending continuing education courses of other associations; or registering for formal education courses in other disciplines. If we believe in optimal health for all people this should be a free exchange without reservation.

To represent dental hygiene with high standards of personal conduct.

Conduct both in the office and in public must be exemplary of professional ideals. Such conduct will not only maintain the image of dentistry as a whole but will aid in elevating its public esteem. It is not necessary to lower standards of attitudes, speech or dress to establish rapport with the patient. Instead, the dental hygienist should be the person the patient will admire and emulate.

Perhaps personal and professional lives should be separated, but in actuality they usually are not. Once a pattern is set it is not difficult nor incompatible to maintain high standards at all times.

Practical Professional Ethics (Examples)

The student's illusion of the ideal and the reality of dental hygiene practice may contrast startlingly in the dental office. Personal and professional ethics cannot be separated, but new situations are met in dental hygiene practice. The dental hygienist must learn to make responsible decisions based on ethical precepts as well as decisions about professional procedures. Unfortunately, compromise is a much-used tool. Professionals' semi-evasive answers are not meant to condone poor dentistry or to "cover-up" for poor care but, rather, to avoid hurting people or the profession unnecessarily. Criticism used as punishment is purely vindictive. Honest criticism should be used to help improve or correct a situation or attitude.

ITEM: The dentist is present in the office, and cannot or will not take time to inspect suspected abnormalities in the patient's mouth. What should the dental hygienist do?

The patient should be rescheduled with an appointment with the dentist. If it is legally permissible, a smear can be made. In any case, a heart-to-heart talk between dentist and dental hygienist is indicated.

ITEM: The patient has an oral lesion which the dental hygienist suspects is a malignancy. The dentist disagrees and does not request the patient to have a biopsy. What is the responsibility of the dental hygienist who strongly believes there should be further examination?

The dentist is legally responsible for all patient care in the office. Does this absolve the dental hygienist from ethical responsibility to the patient? Dental hygiene courses in oral pathology and recognition of abnormalities can be equivalent to that of dental students, and it is possible that the dental hygienist is more cognizant of such problems than a dentist who graduated many years ago. If the dental hygienist is genuinely convinced that the patient needs expert diagnosis then that patient should be urged to seek the care of a qualified specialist. This may appear as employee insubordination, but it also evidences dedication to the precept that patient care is paramount.*

ITEM: Is patient education an ethical responsibility of the dental hygienist?

Yes. By accepting a patient an implied agreement is made to keep his mouth in as healthy a condition as possible. Prophylactic treatment by the dental hygienist loses most of its effectiveness if it is not supplemented by adequate home care. Some patients are knowledgeable about necessary procedures but it is always wise to review them. Extensive restorations may need more than usual care and the dental hygienist should be prepared to advise the patient. It is the dental hygienist's responsibility to tell the patient what home care is needed; it is the patient's responsibility to carry out the instructions.

Professional advice also should include instruction on the need for replacing missing teeth, on correcting poor tongue and swallowing habits or other habits affecting the dentition or facial development, and on the need for orthodontic care. Perhaps more responsibility is involved when a child is the patient, for he is not able to judge his need for care.

The dental hygienist does not diagnose, but does have an ethical responsibility to recognize symptoms of deviations from the normal and bring them to the dentist's attention. In fulfilling the responsibility of providing optimum care the dental hygienist must be able to communicate well with the patient. The method of communication must be suited to the patient's present dental knowledge.

*This is in response to dental hygiene classroom discussion.

ITEM: The patient has had years of regular but not thorough prophylaxis. He now needs periodontal therapy. What is the dental hygienist's responsibility?

The dental hygienist, by law, is not permitted to diagnose the patient's oral condition. The responsibility of the dental hygienist is to inform the dentist of observations made of the patient's teeth and supporting structures. After the dentist evaluates the condition he will outline the procedure to be followed. The patient may be treated in the office, or he may be referred to a specialist. If periodontal patients are treated routinely in the office the procedures to be followed are already known to the dental hygienist. If there is only an occasional periodontal patient treated in the office the dentist no doubt will give explicit directions for treatment.

No matter how this situation is resolved, the patient probably will ask the dental hygienist questions such as: "How did this happen when I had my teeth cleaned regularly?" Is the answer to be that he did not have thorough scaling, that subgingival calculus has been allowed to collect and that perhaps his home care was not adequate? This answer is being critical of the former dentist or dental hygienist, and also of the patient. It may or may not be justified criticism—it would be well to know the facts before condemning. Perhaps the patient's visits were not as regular as he states or perhaps he objected to deep scaling and was allowed to dictate the treatment. Here is an area of ethical responsibility for the dental hygienist, or dentist to explain the consequences of less-than-optimum care. The patient's home care and nutrition usually are far from ideal when all the facts are ascertained. It can be stated that "In this office we believe that it is necessary to your oral health to remove all hard and soft deposits, subgingival as well as supragingival, and to help you learn to keep your mouth clean between office visits."

Assuming that the dental hygienist is to start the treatment, an opportunity is available for patient education about the causes of tissue changes, treatment and what results can be expected, home care and nutritional counseling. If the patient asks why no one told him before, the answer might be that "no person can answer for another, but we want to give our patients the best care that dentistry can currently offer."

ITEM: The patient has dental restorations which need, or will soon need, to be replaced. What is the dental hygienist's obligation?

Remember that the dental hygienist is not to diagnose. Restorations which, in the dental hygienist's judgment, need or will soon need additional care should be recorded for the dentist's information. There is a professional obligation to indicate the present poor condition. No blame needs to be placed on the dentist or the patient; it is merely a restoration which has outlived its usefulness.

The patient should be told that there is a possibility of the need for care, but that the dentist will verify the fact.

The dental hygienist is not legally allowed to diagnose, but is it fair to the patient not to alert him to problem areas? Does it enhance the dental hygienist's intelligence in the patient's eyes to say "I don't know" when the facts are known? At least one legal opinion states that the dental hygienist may tell the patient he has a cavity if it is one that would be obvious to a lay person.*

ITEM: The patient refuses to cooperate in the dental office or in home care. What is the dental hygienist's obligation?

The obligation of the dental hygienist is to make an honest attempt to secure the patient's cooperation in the dental office and motivate him to carry out home care procedures. If he refuses, either verbally or by ignoring these requests, he can be dismissed from the practice. However, he should be told that he needs care, but obviously he can't be helped in this office; thus, he should seek other dental care.

The dental hygienist may feel that it is an ethical responsibility to keep trying to reach the patient for he may not seek other care, and some care is better than total neglect. On the other hand, someone else who is more compatible may be able to establish rapport with the patient and secure his cooperation.

ITEM: The patient asks if he has any cavities, pyorrhea, or malignant lesions. What can the dental hygienist say?

Is the dental hygienist to remain within the law and not diagnose, or does the prime duty to the patient take precedence? Cavities, obvious or suspected, should be charted for the dentist's information and radiographs should be made so that his diagnosis may be based on all possible evidence. Cavities definitely should not be overlooked. Pyorrhea is, in degree, subject to individual judgment. The dental hygienist should be careful in making statements before the dentist talks to the patient.

Many patients are unduly alarmed if mention is made of possible malignant lesions of the oral mucosa. Since microscopic examination is required to verify or disprove the presence of malignancy, it would seem wise to alert the dentist, allowing him to talk to the patient. If the patient asks about some specific area, say that the dentist will examine it.

ITEM: The patient says he has never had his teeth scaled, and asks, "why not?" How can the dental hygienist answer?

How can the dental hygienist know why scaling procedures have not been performed? It is possible that the service had not been offered, but

* State Board of Dental Examiners, California.

perhaps the patient had refused service, or at least did not return for a prophylaxis appointment. Now is the time the benefits of this dental treatment should be explained, assuming that the patient sees the need of treatment and understands how it is performed. The necessity for regular professional and self-care should also be explained.

ITEM: The patient refuses to allow deep scaling because of discomfort, cost or time involved. What should the dental hygienist do?

The dental hygienist's obligation is to attempt to educate the patient about his need for thorough scaling and to motivate him to allow it to be done. If necessary the tissues can be anesthetized by the dentist or dental hygienist, as the state law dictates. If the cost of multiple appointments prohibits treatment or it is a question of time, and the patient cannot be educated to the need for this extensive procedure, either the patient will have to be given compromise care, with his understanding, or he should be requested to secure care in some other office.

ITEM: Does the dental hygienist have an obligation to "practice what you preach" about mouth care and nutrition?

Definitely. The dental hygienist should live up to current standards of the profession, setting an example so patients will be able to see the results of proper care and be motivated to follow instructions relating to themselves. There is no excuse for failing to follow precepts taught to others. Skills and knowledge should be kept current.

ITEM: The patient is a heavy smoker. Does the dental hygienist have an added responsibility to this patient?

It is the obligation of the dental hygienist to give the patient all known facts about smoking, pointing out its deleterious effects on oral tissues as well as the whole body, and encourage the patient to give up this harmful habit. Unless the dental hygienist is a non-smoker, this is an ineffective bit of patient education. Does the dental hygienist have an ethical responsibility to set a good example? Does the dental hygienist have an ethical responsibility at each appointment to urge the patient to change, or is it enough to give him the facts once and then assume he is mature enough to make his own decision on facts presented? Patients can resent repeated criticism to the extent that they will seek another dental office for care. On the other hand, the encouragement of the dental hygienist may be the turning point which could reach the patient and cause him to give up smoking.

ITEM: The dentist requests the dental hygienist to perform a procedure not allowed by law in that jurisdiction. Is the answer "yes" or "no"?

The legal obligation of the dental hygienist is to say "no" and avoid breaking the law. The ethical obligation is a paradox. The dental hygienist is obligated to obey the law and also to follow the directions of the employing dentist and to offer the patient all services compatible with training and skills. The request may be to perform some skill that had been learned which would free the dentist's time and which would give the patient care which might otherwise be postponed. Not performing the procedure may be denying learned capabilities. The individual dental hygienist will have to weigh values of the specific instance and make the decision. No ethical dental hygienist would consider performing any intraoral procedure, legally or illegally, without adequate training and skill.

Experimental programs, in preparation for expanding the duties of the dental hygienist are teaching new procedures. Some states have made legal provision for their performance in dental hygiene practice. Dental hygienists who have been taught these procedure and who move from one type of jurisdiction to another will face new decisions. It is possible that such an act, not sanctioned by law, would be performed for the purpose of testing a law's constitutionality. If the dental hygienist makes this technical violation of the law, it should be an act carefully considered.

ITEM: An unlicensed person is performing intraoral procedures, either with or without the knowledge of the dentist. What is the responsibility of the dental hygienist?

The first obligation, it would seem, would be to talk to the person performing the procedure without legal authority. The dentist, too, should be reminded that he is liable to penalties as well as the involved person. If the procedure is continued, the obligation is to report the action to the state board of dental examiners. Their trained investigators will check the facts and take proper action. The dental hygienist should be very certain before making accusations and must be willing to testify if necessary.

ITEM: An instrument blade is broken and the tip lodges in the patient's mouth. What procedure does the dental hygienist follow?

The patient should be told in a calm manner what has happened. He should be asked not to swallow; his mouth should be rinsed using a pan, not the cuspidor, for rinsings. If the tip is not washed out in this manner, another instrument may be used as an explorer and a knotted section of dental floss can be passed through the embrasure. A radiographic examination should be made to help determine the location of the fragment or to disprove its presence. The dentist, of course, should be told. No admission of liability insurance protection should be made. If there is any possibility of a problem with the patient the insurance company should be notified immediately by telephone, later in writing.

ITEM: Is there ever justification for criticizing the dental treatment performed by another dentist or dental hygienist?

There may be times when criticism is justified, but is the dental hygienist justified in expressing it? No one is perfect and no one is exempt from errors in judgment or performance. Are the exact circumstances under which dental treatment was given known? Is the behavior or attitude of the patient known? Was it emergency treatment intended to be replaced, but the patient didn't return? The patient does not always report accurately. He may have misunderstood the situation or treatment; if in pain he may not have "heard" what he was told; he may try to cover up for his own errors. The patient who comes with a complaint will probably take one with him.

Does the dental hygienist have the right to put another's reputation into jeopardy or to destroy it without knowing all the facts, or to destroy the patient's confidence in the profession? Lest the individual also be judged unfairly, criticism should be used sparingly.

ITEM: The patient insists that the filling which "just fell out" was placed by the dentist. Office records show that the restoration had been done many years before, or perhaps the service was not even performed in this office. What reply does the dental hygienist give?

This is not exactly the dental hygienist's problem but, being a buffer between the patient and the dentist, the question is often asked and must be answered. Make a statement based on the records of the patient. There may be no way to convince the patient that he is wrong; he may remain sure that the records are in error. Arguing with him is poor policy. The dentist should be alerted to the situation before he sees the patient and will have to decide whether he will replace the filling without charge, or replace it for a fee which he will have to arrange with the patient.

ITEM: The patient says his former dentist, or an oral surgeon, "pulled" the wrong tooth, or that a perfectly good tooth was extracted. What statement should the dental hygienist make?

Instructions can be written incorrectly, misread or misinterpreted. There is very little that should be said. If this was a very recent extraction the patient may be looking for an opinion to support a law suit. The answer then should be that not knowing anything about the case there is no basis for an opinion. If this is an extraction done many years before and it truly was an error, it was a regrettable one.

Keep in mind that facts are not known and patients can be wrong, too. A perfectly good tooth may not have had hard or soft tissue support.

ITEM: The patient says he was overcharged in another office, perhaps quoting the fee, and asks for an opinion. Should the dental hygienist express an opinion?

The only explanation to the question of fees is that fees do vary according to the area of practice and the overhead expenses of the office, and only the dentist himself knows the basis for his fees. Fees should be discussed with the person who decides them. If fees in one office are lower than those in a former office the patient probably will not complain; hopefully, he will not consider the care to be inferior. Higher fees will have to be justified, and overhead expenses should not be the prime selling point. Standards of care should never be lowered in order to reduce costs. The dental hygienist could indicate that this is the best care, the best treatment or restoration that the office staff can give, and is the same care which is given to the dentist's family, and the fee for this type of care is fair.

It is better not to know fees charged by the specialists, for such fees are based on the individual care needed and each case is different. The patient should understand that he is paying for the special knowledge and skill possessed by the operator to provide treatment for his problem.

ITEM: The patient asserts that a filling was defective because the tooth has now decayed. How can the dental hygienist explain this?

Can the dental hygienist actually tell by looking at the tooth, or the radiographs, that the cause of decay was faulty workmanship? Of course not. It is better to explain the causes of secondary decay and include the fact that 90% of the durability of dental restorations depends on the patient's daily care. Since living tissues and people are involved there can be no guarantee of the life of restorations, for the dentist has no control over outside factors.

Office Procedures

The employment interview should disclose certain routine office procedures, or lack of them. The use of radiographic examinations and health histories, the length of prophylaxis appointments and sterile techniques are easily determined. Such things as the quality of services are not usually known except through experience. To reject employment will avoid some problems but others will be met in practice, for there is no guarantee of complete follow-through on stated procedures.

The fact that another professionally trained person routinely sees completed dental restorations stimulates the average dentist to do his best. The dentist who knowingly gives inferior service is not likely to employ a dental hygienist. Some of the following statements are more hypothetical than real but they may stimulate discussion and encourage personal ethical actions.

ITEM: How should remuneration of the dental hygienist be determined?

Salary, commission or a combination of the two methods are all acceptable means of determining the type of reimbursement of the dental hygienist, and that choice and the amount are made through agreement between the dentist and dental hygienist.

The dental hygienist is an employee, not a separate entity, and a daily or weekly salary enhances the philosophy of being a team member in the dental office. When the dental hygienist performs a variety of functions in addition to the traditional oral prophylaxis, salary is the practical method of reimbursement. The quality and quantity of patient services should be determined by the ethics of the dentist and dental hygienist rather than by the type or amount of compensation.

Only by being an asset to the office can an increase in remuneration be justified. If that can be documented, then state the facts and make a reasonable request. It is not wrong to acknowledge capabilities as well as increased living costs, but do not over-rate them. If improvement in some areas of work is needed, establish criteria to be met within a specified time limit and arrange for another review.

When agreements are reached it is good business practice to write a memo in duplicate outlining the points agreed upon, for everyone tends to forget some things.

ITEM: Dental office procedures do not require health histories.

Health histories are a legal and a physical protection to all persons involved. Even though the patient may not give honest or complete answers to health history questions, an attempt has been made to determine illnesses and allergic reactions which could make dental treatment hazardous to the patient or the operator. Legal responsibility for poor results is thus avoided. There is an ethical responsibility to the patient to avoid harming him. As examples, bleeding caused by prophylactic instrumentation can release harmful bacteria into the bloodstream and damage a rheumatic heart. If the facts are known, the patient can be premedicated with the antibiotic of choice and procedures performed without danger. The patient with hepatitis can be an infectious hazard to the operator and potentially to other patients.

The dental hygienist has two choices. An explanation to the dentist-employer might persuade him to include the necessary procedure in the office routine or to allow the dental hygienist to use a health history for all oral prophylaxis patients. The use of health histories by the dental hygienist might be a means to prove their worth and institute their regular use. If the dentist rejects the use of health histories altogether the dental hygienist must decide whether it is possible to work taking chances with the health of the patient and self, or whether it is better to seek other employment.

ITEM: Dental office procedures do not require radiographic surveys.

Radiographs are necessary diagnostic aids as well as legal evidence of existing conditions. Their use shows the intent of the dentist to offer the patient complete service.

If office policy does not include complete radiographic surveys of new patients and routine radiographic surveys of recall patients, the dental hygienist may try to persuade the dentist to follow this procedure. If the attempt is unsuccessful, the decision must be made to remain under existing conditions or find other employment. Can the dental hygienist condone not giving the patient the benefit of all diagnostic aids possible?

ITEM: Dental office staff members do not follow accepted sterilizing techniques.

It is difficult to imagine that today's dentist does not use accepted sterilizing techniques because of the common knowledge of danger of transmitting infections. Sanitizing procedures, however, can be lax or overlooked and the dental hygienist can insist on proper care in the assigned operatory. Other office personnel can be persuaded to use better procedures.

ITEM: Dental office policy is to schedule patients on short appointments which do not allow the dental hygienist adequate time for prophylaxis procedures and instruction in home care and nutrition.

If employment is accepted with knowledge of this general office policy, the dental hygienist should give thought to personal values and motives. Too often short appointments mean more income for the office for an esthetic procedure rather than a preventive treatment and patient education. Short appointments with frequent recall patients may be acceptable. The dental hygienist must evaluate the situation and decide whether or not patients' needs are being met. Length and frequency of appointments should be flexible and based on the needs of the individual patient. Appointments should be determined by the dental hygienist in keeping with the dentist's policy.

ITEM: Incipient caries are ignored.

What is the meaning of "incipient" caries? To some dentists any initial carious lesion should be restored at once. To others it is an area to be watched. These dentists believe that if the patient's decay rate and home care habits are known, and that if the patient will return for regular inspections, restoration of these areas can be delayed. There may be a lapse of years before active decay is evident, but there is no time guarantee, and many dentists treat any degree of decay. If restoration is postponed, the patient should be told of the condition and its possibilities. The explanation might be part of the dental hygienist's patient education.

ITEM: Must recall notices be sent to undesirable patients?

What is an "undesirable" patient—one whose personality clashes with the dentist's, one who neglects home care, one who is slow in paying incurred bills, or one who is handicapped in some manner? Each of these various personalities is entitled to dental care, especially when he has voluntarily sought care. It is the ethical responsibility of the dental hygienist to send reminders, unless asked not to do so, and to make an honest effort in patient education. Patients change, too, and many will respond when real concern is shown.

ITEM: The dental hygienist is leaving the dental office for another. Can notices be sent to patients informing them of the change?

These are the dentist's patients, not the dental hygienist's. Though patients may choose the dentist and dental hygienist who give them dental care, it is not acceptable to ask them to make a change. If the dental hygienist is leaving because of substandard dental procedures being performed and believes there is a responsibility to inform patients of this, serious thought should be given to the situation before making statements. Is the dental hygienist competent to judge the dentist's work? Is the judgment based on fact or personal opinion?

ITEM: The dental hygienist is terminating employment. How much notice should be given?

A minimum of two weeks' notice should be given the dentist, but a month's notice is better. It is often difficult to secure a replacement. If patients are appointed in advance, the responsible dental hygienist would not want to leave them without care, nor leave the dentist in a difficult position. Irresponsible resignations reflect adversely on the entire profession of dental hygiene. If a position is accepted with the knowledge that it is only for six months or a year, the dental hygienist should inform the dentist of this stipulation.

Dental Dilemmas

ITEM: Is there an obligation to perform "ideal" dentistry or can there be an ethical compromise?

To answer this question adequately "ideal dentistry" needs to be defined. Complete reconstruction may be ideal in the sense that it would be the best means of restoring the patient's mouth to a healthy, functional and esthetic entity. For the patient whose finances will not permit or justify this extensive procedure, silver amalgam restorations which arrest decay and restore teeth to function may prove to be an ethical compromise. The dentist should not make the decision for the patient. Instead, the ideal procedure should be outlined but alternatives can be offered. Adequate patient education may influence the decision, but it is as unethical to persuade the patient to spend a large sum of money on himself if it means denying his family necessary items as it would be to neglect him altogether. If total dentistry is not accomplished, the dental hygienist can follow up in subsequent prophylaxis appointments and encourage the patient to complete the work at some future time.

ITEM: Can the patient ever dictate his own treatment?

The patient may choose from alternate treatment plans, such as gold inlays or silver amalgam restorations, extraction or no extraction, treatment or no treatment. The dentist is obligated to inform the patient of what he believes is needed and why such treatment is needed, but he is never obligated to perform any dental operation contrary to his professional judgment.

ITEM: Patient confidences are to be respected. Are there any exceptions?

Personal confidences and health histories are to be respected. In discussing case histories with professional colleagues nothing should be said which would identify an individual. Exceptions to the rule of confidence are patients with syphilis and tuberculosis, which must be reported to the proper authorities. This is a legal and an ethical responsibility.

References

Code of Ethics, ADHA. 1926, 1962, 1969.

Gurley, John E.: *Professional Ethics in Dentistry.* St. Louis, College of Dentists, 1961.

Lillie, William: *An Introduction to Ethics.* 3rd ed. New York, Barnes & Noble, 1961.

Lovett, Ethelbert: *An Approach to Ethics.* Baltimore, Waverly Press, Inc., 1963.

Chapter 3

Responsibilities of the Dental Hygienist

General Responsibilities of Citizenship

"Every profession," George Bernard Shaw, novelist, playwright and Nobel Prize winner in literature, once remarked in a usual half-truth, "is a conspiracy against the laity." Conspiracy or not, professions are as characteristic of modern society as crafts were of ancient societies. A phenomenon of all highly industrialized and urbanized societies, the "professionals" per 100,000 population in the United States increased from 859 in 1870 to 3310 in 1950.

For the profession that is dental hygiene, knowledge and skill go hand-in-hand. Its responsibility is to control the balance between the system and the concerns of the individual as both a biological organism and a personality complex. Health is a major consideration of normal social participation; incapacity for such participation is a central criterion of illness; safeguarding health and controlling physical processes constitute social interests.

Because dental hygiene has persuasively shown that it is the master of its special craft, society has been willing to grant the profession the right of licensure. Licensure validates the adequacy of the dental hygienist's education and competence. The profession of dental hygiene offers unique services not available elsewhere, and in its operational dynamics the profession does not rely upon the passive action of market forces.

The problems encountered in dental offices are those which the patient cannot solve but can be solved by the dentist and dental hygienist. Usually the patient does not choose the dental hygienist by a measurable criterion of competence. When the service is completed, the patient usually is not competent to judge if it was properly done. The highest rewards of prestige and remuneration are obtained by the dental hygienist who meets and exceeds professional role obligations.

As a professional, the dental hygienist expects to apply knowledge to the problems of a patient. Scientifically, the dental hygienist knows aspects of biological and physical sciences; culturally, the professional applies knowledge of behavioral disciplines. The dental hygienist pursues knowledge in order to improve practice. Day-by-day dental hygiene practice requires more specialized education for, as dentistry advances, more specialized knowledge is needed and dentists increasingly delegate more technical functions to dental hygienists.

It has been stated that dental hygiene is not a stepping stone to another profession; rather, it is a separate endeavor with specific objectives. Since it is based upon well established scientific principles of preventive dentistry, dental hygiene has attempted to satisfy that indispensable social need, the need for dental health. However, with the expansion of services a reality today, the upward mobility of the profession is a valid goal and the dental hygienist must not be hemmed in by rigid boundaries of prejudice or current practice limitations. Possession of a body of specialized and systematized knowledge and clinical educational and social skills can allow the dental hygienist to provide needed care and thus release the dentist's time to offer diagnostic and more technical operative services to an ever-increasing number of people.

For a calling to attain the dignity and distinction of a profession it must have certain moral values. One value is helping to build a better life for people. The modern graduate is cognizant of responsibility for dental health of office patients as well as non-patients within the community. Dental practice changes with the nature and demands of our society. Today's dental practice includes people in hospitals and homes for the chronically ill and aged. To continue to provide dental care for regular patients and to add the increasing numbers of patients who participate in dental insurance plans, especially children who qualify under federal health insurance funds, professional productivity must be increased.

To assist in meeting these demands, dental hygienists must accept and assume greater responsibility for increasing the numbers of qualified auxiliary personnel to work with dentistry in providing service. These new demands on dental hygiene will add other dimensions to the responsibilities assumed by this professional dental health auxiliary.

Where science advances knowledge, dental hygiene applies this knowledge. Conceived and founded on the premise that oral hygiene is important for dental health, dental hygienists' moral values include responsibilities for dental hygiene education. Performing clinical, educational and community services, the dental hygienist works in a spectrum extending from general and specialty dental offices to public health agencies, from schools to hospitals, from industrial organizations to the armed forces.

Today, scientists are facing the challenge of the unknown. While inventive minds are testing methods of sophisticated space exploration, investigators are probing the world of microorganisms hoping to eliminate what have seemed to be inevitable disease processes. Dental hygiene, too, is facing the challenge of the unknown. That which has previously been accepted as dental hygiene practice will no longer suffice for today's philosophy of dentistry. In order to survive, dental hygiene must explore recognized gaps in the world of dentistry and general health. Dental hygienists must help ascertain what is to be done to make optimal health available to everyone, and they must become involved intimately in providing motivation and education as well as service. There are unlimited opportunities for service in the dental health field waiting to be discovered and used. Providing these services can aid in making the expectations of a better, healthier future a reality for those who have never enjoyed such benefits, and can contribute to the self-realization which comes when one gives of himself freely and gladly.

As the differentiation of American society has increased, and problems of inclusion and upgrading have become particularly important, the legal definition of rights and responsibilities has gained in importance. Simultaneously, in this era of developing technology and exploding population, the relationships of dental hygiene to the community-at-large is of crucial consideration. With an expanding clientele, the dental hygienist must not assume so many functions that existing professional standards will be jeopardized.

Dental hygienists must become acutely aware of socio-economic problems facing the world, and the profession in particular, and they must be willing and prepared for a more significant contribution in delivering health services. The dental hygienist who can draw upon a rational approach and fund of learning to help reshape dental care delivery in an expanding population will make a tremendous contribution to American society.

Society needs the vital talents of the dental hygienist whose moral values include a long-term effort to make resources meet needs. The dental hygienist should reach beyond an inner circle of personal interest, resist adversity, and stay on the job until it is done. The dental hygienist never strays far from pragmatism for ideas are constantly tested by action. Yet, there is no freedom to stagnate, to live without dreams, to have no greater aim than a commitment to profit and pleasure alone.

In terms of sheer material potency and well-being, members of the profession live in an era without equal or precedent. American society, despite its flaws and blemishes, has no equal in human history for scope, opportunity and earning power. While material well-being may not be the first and certainly is not the only requirement for happiness, it surely helps.

Man does not live by bread alone, but neither can he live without it. In keeping with more responsible functions, the dental hygienist earns a measure of independence, prestige and financial security.

For dental hygienists the challenge of our faith, the true crisis of our time, lies at a deeper level. The goal of life is more than material advancement; it is the triumph of spirit over matter. The hallmark of this profession is good deeds—good deeds inspired by a concern for human values and dedicated to a respect for the dignity and worth of mankind.

Idealism in modern times is not always fashionable. Unless something can be justified by hard-headed self-interest, it is said to have "no chance." But it should be remembered that kindness and idealism may be practical too and, practical or not, they stand well in the eyes of God. The highest purpose of dental hygiene is to serve not just our selfish aims, but the cause of mankind.

This is an age in which so many mentors of the public mind—from psychiatrists to advertisers—speak in terms of "what we owe ourselves." Dental hygienists, as educated and privileged people, have a broad responsibility to protect and improve what they have inherited and what they must preserve. The dental hygienist, by virtue of public and private position, the role in the family and community, the prospects for the future and the legacy from the past, must be more responsible than many other Americans. Increased functions beget increased responsibilities, for "of those to whom much is given, much is required." Participating in dental hygiene requires an attitude, a moral view and a willingness to assume day-to-day responsibilities in areas of leadership, education and service.

Responsibilities of Leadership

Amid the genius, violence, crime and wealth of Renaissance Italy, Niccolo Machiavelli, a Florentine diplomat and an ardent advocate of the image of the mindless mass and the strong-willed leader, wrote:

> And it must be understood that a Prince . . . . cannot observe all those things which are considered good in men, being often obligated . . . . to act against faith, against charity, against humanity.

The Machiavellian concept of leadership is obsolete in urban, industrial America. Leadership can no longer be viewed as a fixed set of traits and attributes, biologically peculiar to some individuals, and there can be no dependence on concepts applying to the elite, to autocratic systems, or to rigid classes and castes.

Leadership in dental hygiene has necessarily become the shared responsibility of all in the pursuit of common and compatible goals. Leadership today is a characteristic of the total profession rather than of individuals or individual acts. All members have relevant abilities, resources and personal characteristics, and these, combined with functional needs of the profession, determine the role that the individual member enacts. Because of the increasing complexity of dental health problems of the world, many persons with highly technical and administrative expertise are required to assume exceptional leadership roles in the profession. Since leadership is a complex social function rather than simply a property of an individual, all dental hygienists must lead to some degree. The same member may manifest different degrees of leadership behavior—being a leader only at one point in time, or a leader relative only to certain areas of collective action. The leader must be identified with the most pervasive goals of the profession—values that must be expressed and epitomized. Dental hygienist leaders must bridge the social and political distance between professional knowledge and the need for public responsiveness.

The role of dental hygienists in the family and the community, the public and private position, the prospects for the future and the legacy from the past—all of these define areas of "need" for leadership.

The headlines of today are the heritage of yesterday. In 1973 there were more than two hundred ten million Americans, including more than one hundred thousand dentists and about twenty thousand practicing dental hygienists. In a given year, no more than half the population sees a dentist. With a growing population expressing a greater demand for health services, including dentistry; with federal health legislation, especially for the medically indigent; with the extension of the practice of dentistry to people in institutions, hospitals and homes for the chronically ill and aged; with the mushrooming growth of dental insurance and prepayment programs; with the American Dental Association's "National Dental Health Program for Children"—with all of these the long-forecast shortage of dental manpower has become a reality.

The general practice of dentistry is extending beyond the four walls of the operatory. Since 1960 approximately 40 per cent of the accredited dental schools in the United States have established departments of community or social dentistry. Educational and preventive procedures are significant parts of modern dental practice. Today, against the background of a shortage of manpower and changing treatment demands, many dentists are increasing their productivity through the efficient use of auxiliary personnel. Dental hygiene has helped and can help dentistry meet further needs of modern-day society where the public attitude is that health is a right and not a privilege.

This age will have to be marked by innovation and daring to meet unprecedented problems with intelligent solutions. Dentistry and dental hygiene are engaged in a long-term effort to make resources meet society's needs. For this age of specialization, it might seem that dental hygienists, educated and licensed in the fields of prevention, education and therapeutics, should not be diverted to restorative services, and that any expansion of duties for the dental hygienist at this time should increase the scope and depth of preventive and educational services related to periodontal disease. But the restorative services a dental hygienist might perform should not be overlooked in the reassignment of duties of auxiliary personnel. Formal educational programs and licensing procedures already established would facilitate needed additional training for extended functions in the restorative field of dentistry.

However, fundamental decisions must be made, decisions which will need to be supported by facts not presently available. Adequate studies need to be carried out on the extension of duties of the dental hygienist, and careful evaluation of data must be made before it can be determined which additional duties can be assigned to the dental hygienist and which could be assigned to another dental auxiliary to maintain the highest efficiency in office or clinic.

Reallocation of procedures will have to be accompanied by practice act revisions and new board regulations. Here are fertile fields in which dental hygienists must work constructively and cooperatively with dentistry. Many states have modernized their dental practice acts delegating more services to auxiliaries. It is generally agreed that practice acts should be broad statements, permissive in nature rather than restrictive. In the last analysis, utilization of the educated dental hygienist's extended functions is the key to meeting the need.

With thousands of dollars available or already invested in facilities and equipment, schools of dental hygiene are developing at a faster rate than the profession's ability to prepare qualified dental hygiene teachers and administrators. Today, dental schools are placing greater emphasis on preventive dentistry and community health. Today's and tomorrow's graduates of these schools know what skills and abilities the dental hygienist should possess.

The dental hygienist must share professional skills and knowledge with all segments of the public. By participating in community programs, in keeping with the dignity of the profession and appropriate to the situation, the dental hygienist demonstrates leadership and assistance in improving the health of others.

Leaders are not always born; most of them are self-made. One common attribute is fluent communication. A leader knows what is going on about him, is aware of the concerns of the people with whom he works, and knows how they will be affected when decisions are made.

Responsibilities of Education

Education is the keystone in the arch of progress. Clark Kerr, former President of the University of California, predicted in 1963 that soon the "knowledge" industry will occupy the key role in the American economy occupied by the railroad industry a hundred years ago. In the last ten years mankind has acquired more scientific information than in all previous history. Accelerating change is the one universal human prospect and, in the process, the human mind never can be legislated out of its curiosity and constant inquiry for new truths. More than ever before, education has become a continuous, lifelong process. If the complex demands of society are to be met, an increasing proportion of time must be spent in continuing the dental hygienist's education. "Every five years one relearns his vocation—or learns a substitute, new vocation and time intervals will become shorter as automation increases."* The profession has reached the plateau where formal education is only the beginning of a lifelong learning process.

In a time of turbulence and change, knowledge is power; only by applying true understanding and good judgment are current challenges mastered. The dental hygienist must strive to acquire knowledge—and to temper this knowledge with wisdom. With a compassionate eye and a deft hand, the dental hygienist can treat each individual fairly and justly.

It has been said that the best things in life are free. Paradoxically we pay, contributing money, time and energy, for all we receive. But "best" in its finest sense identifies ephemeral emotional characteristics which make man a reasoning creature. Foremost among these qualities are concern for others, recognition and acceptance of the need for involvement in life, and an insatiable curiosity about the world and its people which makes man eager to learn as long as he has life.

The problems of today must not be allowed to overshadow the possibilities of tomorrow. Too many dental hygienists in the past have accepted the profession as a stop-gap between school and marriage, rather than their life's work. No longer can a commitment to service be ignored; there must be a return to the public. Skills constantly must be improved and increased to aid in delivering health care. Dental hygienists are motivated by the desire to provide a health service; presumably they are altruistic and their pleasure comes from the rewarding feeling of making significant contributions to the health and happiness of someone else. However, they must explore their talents fully and share them freely.

Today, science and technology are becoming major parts of the creative and cultural activities of man. There is an ascending interest in the work of science and a demand for information by the public at a higher and higher level of literacy, authenticity and authority. The dental hygienist has an important and continuing responsibility to increase knowledge and skill and to communicate effectively with all segments of the population.

Scientific and technological advances in dentistry demand that the dental hygienist be aware of and use new scientific discoveries. It is the dental hygienist's responsibility to apply scientific knowledge and to motivate the public. For example, preventive dentistry emphasizes oral hygiene, adequate nutrition including dietary restriction of certain sugars, fluoridation

* Tondow, Murray: In *Man-Machine System in Education* (Loughary, John W., Ed.) New York, Harper and Row, 1966.

and topical applications of fluorides. Increasing public utilization of orthodontics and restorative dental services as preventive measures is as important to the dental hygienist as research methods are to the scientist.

Subjects such as English and speech should be of more than academic interest to the dental hygienist for this knowledge aids and guides the professional's relationships with patients and office personnel. The public assumes that the professional person has specific knowledge of his field, but these skills will allow the practitioner to communicate with his public.

The dental hygienist with basic knowledge of psychology can learn to make a primary evaluation of the patient's personality and attitude toward dental health. Sociologic principles assist the dental hygienist in dealing with the individual as a member of his community as well as with specific groups in a larger community. It is the shared knowledge of other professions and disciplines that has enabled dental hygienists to recognize patients as social as well as biological beings.

Physical sciences supply reasons, logic and explanations for technical procedures, forming a foundation for the clinical practice of dental hygiene. The ability of the dental hygienist to evaluate the patient's physical and dental health needs is acquired through knowledge of pathology, microbiology, anatomy, physiology, and biochemistry. All these needs, psychological, physical and social, must be evaluated accurately by the practitioner before services can be planned or administered. Currently, there is no substitute for formal education in these basic disciplines.

Responsibilities to the Community

Presently there is a trend toward more activity, more responsibility, more involvement in community affairs. The dental hygienist cannot be content to ask "why" when "why not" will broaden the base of contribution to society.

When the dental hygienist begins to fulfill responsibilities to the community, the obligations of a responsible citizen are assumed. Civic duties include being an informed, intelligent voter and a law-abiding individual.

Recent events, such as legislative activity, strongly suggest a significant lack of knowledge and understanding in the public mind about the dental and scientific communities. Dental hygienists must continue to try to establish, assist and encourage a beneficial rapport with the public in order to stimulate a deeper interest and confidence in the achievements of dentistry and dental hygiene.

In addition, the dental hygienist should give freely of skills and knowledge in the field of dental health in such activity areas as health departments, schools, fluoridation campaigns, service clubs and youth groups, performing clinically, motivating the public toward achieving better oral and general health. Appearance on radio or television programs promoting dental health in accordance with accepted professional standards, writing articles for publication and counselling students about the profession are other ways of fulfilling responsibilities to the community. In some manner, dental hygienists must be adhesive and cohesive forces in this galaxy of opportunities.

Responsibilities of Service

Patient

The average person does not speculate about the separation of duties and responsibilities of the dental health team. The average person simplifies and personifies dentistry, and the profession takes its coloration for him from the acts of all. Both dentists and dental auxiliaries have, therefore, a responsibility for the picture that emerges. Anyone can mar it. Since the dental hygienist may represent the entire profession to the patient, each one must not only exemplify the traits which the public holds as objectives but improve the professional image as it is accepted today.

The average person assumes that communication is a natural phenomenon but communication is effective only when some thought is given to it. In order to have meaningful contact one must first of all respect others as individuals. Communication is what is said, how it is said and what effect it has on the listener. Clarity and honesty of expression and ability to influence people are all important parts of the process. Often, too much is assumed by the speaker, for the assumptive worlds of people are not the same. That is, words have different meanings for various people and hearing and listening may differ. The dental hygienist, to communicate effectively, must learn to recognize total meaning and then respond appropriately to explicit and implicit feelings of others.

Much significant communication is non-verbal, that is, the listener conveys thoughts and attitudes through posture, facial expressions, gestures and physical movements. Looking at the ceiling, sighing, shifting to turn away, frowning, smiling or nodding are conscious or unconscious communications between the dental hygienist and another person.

A new patient is influenced first of all by appearances of the office and staff, or by the voice that answers his telephone call. The office should reflect the attitudes of those who work within it. Personal appearance of the dentist and all auxiliaries, not only in dress but in attitudes demonstrated in face, voice and manner, should be cultivated to express the high ideals and motives of the profession. Nothing is more inexpensive than a warm smile on the face and in the voice.

All the clinical services of the dental hygienist must be directed to the patient in order to fulfill the commitment to aid individuals attain and maintain optimum oral health. Total dental health care requires variations in procedures to meet the diverse needs of individuals. Often, since the patient's first appointment is with the dental hygienist, she must assume responsibility for projecting a favorable opinion of the office and its personnel. On a patient's first visit he is concerned primarily with personalities in the office and the possibility of needing major dental work. Professional advice about preventive home procedures will fall very likely on deaf ears. The dental hygienist needs to be sensitive to the patient's motivation for responding.

Accurate data through a comprehensive health history, oral inspection and its recording, and a comprehensive radiographic survey should be compiled for the patient's welfare and for the dentist's information. The dental hygienist needs to gather this data accurately but without alarming or embarrassing the patient at any time. Radiographs are a necessary part of the complete oral survey and health history. It is the dental hygienist's responsibility to expose films properly, understand adequate radiographic hygiene practices, and interpret the films for scaling procedures and any other purposes legally accepted in the place of practice.

While performing a thorough oral examination, scaling and polishing the teeth, the dental hygienist must manage to stimulate the patient's personal responsibility for home care, explaining toothbrushing and auxiliary methods of stimulation and cleansing, and the value of good nutrition. Dental prophylaxis and all means of disease prevention are topics within the scope of the dental hygienist's responsibility to the patient.

Oral health instruction should be given according to the wishes of the dentist, and the dental hygienist should be prepared to answer questions concerning many dental problems related to present conditions, proposed treatment and future care. The main responsibility for treatment lies with the dentist, but questions often are directed to the dental hygienist during the oral prophylaxis appointment.

Basic needs or drives for achievement, independence, belonging, love, recognition and self-esteem are individual urges the dental hygienist will need to consider in identifying motivation of the patient to return for preventive recall care. There are three basic principles underlying a workable recall system: motivating the patient, and positive appointment and reappointment systems. The mechanics of the recall may be carried out by the same person or another auxiliary in the office.

Alumnae

For the graduate of a dental hygiene program within a dental school there is a responsibility to the school. The alumnae group provides liaison between the school and its graduates and provides a group which can be very influential in the growth and development of the school. This can be growth in expanding the physical facilities so that more students can be accommodated, upgrading and increasing the equipment or teaching methods or aids of the program, recruitment of qualified students or development of continuing education courses. Dental hygienists should accept their responsibility and contribute in some manner, financially or physically, to their alumnae association to assure the continuance of the educational status of dental hygiene and so that the image of dental hygiene will be further increased in the eyes of the public. Alumnae meetings offer one more opportunity to increase and share knowledge and skills.

Self

Confucius is credited with saying "A picture is worth a thousand words." If this is true, then the dental hygienist who presents an accurate image of the ideal personification of the profession has made a good beginning. The dental hygienist has a particular role in society, not only to care for people but to care about people. The public has rather specific expectations for dental personnel, so in choosing dental hygiene as a career certain obligations must be met during professional working hours. A professional appearance is the result of good health and good grooming. Personal and oral health are primary responsibilities of the dental hygienist who demonstrates an example and speaks with authority. Mental health indicating emotional maturity will inspire confidence and will reflect favorably in all phases of the dental hygienist's duties and contributions to professional and community activities. A zest for life, evidenced by enthusiasm for everyday office confrontations, is contagious and impressive.

Respect for oneself demonstrated by professional appearance and demeanor indicates to the patient the respect he will receive from the operator. Careless attire and grooming may indicate that the operator also may neglect the patient's welfare. Through example the professional most effectively encourages improvement in the patient's appearance and attitudes.

In spite of marked changes in personal attire, the desirable qualities of cleanliness, neatness and attractiveness have not changed. Cleanliness is still next to Godliness for the dental hygienist whose person must be immaculate, whose uniform must be fresh, becoming and reasonable in style, whose hair style must be neat, and whose shoes must be clean as well as comfortable. The lavender-banded cap is the distinctive insignia of the dental hygienist and for years has been worn with pride. Today's dental hygienist lives in a world of rapidly changing traditions and independent thinking and does not always follow this custom. The white cap may indicate servitude to some and does not complement the colored or pants uniform of others. It might be argued that unless all female members of the oral health team wear caps no member should be given particular identification. In any case, since there are now many males in the profession, it is obvious that not all dental hygienists will wear caps.

Contemporary mores allow more latitude in the manner of dress in the professional office than in former years but certain basic principles still apply. Just as the dental office is no longer severely starkly white from walls to basic equipment, the conventional white uniform, still acceptable, is now being replaced in many offices with color, in the belief that the patient is more relaxed in an informal atmosphere. For the dental hygienist who works from a seated position, culottes can be an acceptable compromise to shorter skirts. Pant-suit uniforms are acceptable in most offices.

The dental hygienist's hands must be well groomed, with short fingernails. The face, so close to the patient's eyes, can be enhanced with make-up in moderation and good taste. Extreme hair styles should be reserved for after office hours, as should bright nail polish. For the male dental hygienist well-groomed hair and face, conforming to acceptable office standards, are essential.

Glasses should be worn as protection from flying debris which can cause eye infection or loss of sight. Jewelry should be confined to a watch and a wedding band for there is danger of damage from water, mercury, or office medicaments in addition to the facts that jewelry can be distracting to the patient and is a potential breeding place for bacteria. All one need do is inspect microscopically a ring worn while hands are thoroughly scrubbed and dried. The ring is still covered with huge mountains of debris and bacteria.

It is wise to have duplicate uniform items in reserve for emergencies which occasionally arise. All articles of clothing need to be checked frequently and kept in good repair or replaced. To wonder whether any part of the uniform is "clean enough" is positive proof that it isn't.

Street clothes are preferable for street wear, and the cap is never worn outside the professional environment. Seeing a dental hygienist in a restaurant in uniform is comparable to seeing the gowned surgeon at a tea party. The professional wears a uniform to protect the patient, not to protect his own street clothes.

Discretion and judgment in personal and professional actions are attributes of the dental hygienist. Desirable personal qualities can be cultivated so the individual will be known as a gracious, warm, sincere person who is tactful and intuitive in all situations. Inherently alert, curious and adaptive, the dental hygienist can utilize these traits to achieve increased creativity. It is a fact that the storage power of the brain is inexhaustible, and the more it stores the more capacity it gains. By being receptive to new ideas, continually acquiring new facts and opinions and learning to sort ideas logically, a pleasing personality will be developed and expanded.

Dentist and His Office

Each member of the office staff is expected to assume a multitude of responsibilities. Acceptance and fulfillment of these responsibilities are vital to the efficiency and cooperative atmosphere of the office. The dental hygienist must be willing to assume responsibilities allocated by the individual dentist and the profession and must fulfill them with a spirit of cheerful cooperation. In a large dental practice, or in clinics, the dental hygienist's duties are usually limited to oral prophylaxis, patient education, radiographic surveys and supervising the recall system. However, duties of other staff members should be learned so that problems are better understood and assistance may be given as needed. In a one- or two-auxiliary office it is mandatory that the dental hygienist be familiar with all procedures so that continuity of operation and patient services will not be disrupted because of illness or emergency.

Good interpersonal relationships take respect, cooperation and understanding within the group. Personal and professional acceptance must be earned by each member of the dental team. The fact that money, time and effort have been invested in dental hygiene training should not be allowed to create a "self-opinion" out of proportion to real value. Security and a fair monetary return can be expected, but the individual must be sure that he is worthy. Money should be the return for effort, not the goal. In offices where mutual confidence and respect exist the patient enters a comfortable and professional environment. Because the attitude of the dental hygienist toward the employer and other staff members affects the efficiency of all, there should be obvious pride and faith in the work of the employer and other personnel. The dental hygienist must have confidence as well in personal abilities and competence. Attendance at continuing education courses and scientific sessions and active participation in professional and community affairs are prerequisites to ability, confidence and competence.

Cooperation and understanding will be augmented if office policies are respected by all personnel. Normal responsibilities include observance of office hours and scheduling of appointments, promptness, assisting other staff members, and knowing what the dentist expects and making every effort to perform at or above his expectations. The dental hygienist who adapts to people and circumstances and is dependable, enthusiastic and tactful is an asset to the dentist, his practice and the profession.

Loyalty is expected from the dental hygienist—loyalty to the dentist as a person and to the office as a functioning unit. Individual patients, their dental treatment and fees are not discussed with outsiders. The patient and dentist have every right to expect the confidence of their personal matters to be observed. The dental hygienist who becomes known as an "office hopper" is not manifesting the loyalty which should be given to the employing dentist. If it is necessary to make a change, adequate notice should be given so the dentist is not left with confirmed appointments which cannot be honored and patients are not denied the care they are entitled to expect.

Profession

In 1776 a small group of Americans drafted a document that is still valid and quotable; although short, it is succinct. In part, it reads: "We hold these truths to be self-evident; that all men are created equal; that they are endowed by their Creator with certain inalienable rights; that among them are life, liberty and the pursuit of happiness." Despite the basic truth of this statement, equality of abilities is not a fact and more is expected of the professional person than of others. In addition to community service the dental hygienist has a very definite commitment to the profession, an obligation to assist in improvement of public opinion of dentistry and dental hygiene. Belief in the profession and enthusiasm for its many possibilities for service to people should make the dental hygienist a constant recruiter of qualified individuals into the profession.

Membership in the professional organizations is not just a responsibility and obligation of the dental hygienist. It is insurance for the protection and improvement of the profession's future. Although active support is most desirable, moral and financial support are acceptable alternatives. An individual's participation as an officer, committee member, clinician, speaker or voting member is vital to the survival of the profession's collective voice.

The duties of any active, participating member are demanding and time consuming but the rewards outweigh these impediments. Dental hygienists with leadership qualities, and those who desire to develop them, as well as those who are concerned and want to share in directing the future of their profession, should volunteer to serve. Another necessary activity is preparing material for publication, for one way in which a profession grows is through research and communication.

Each member of the profession should be informed about legislation affecting dental hygiene, changes in dental practice acts and trends in the delivery of dental care. Organized dental hygienists should work cooperatively and intelligently to create and support favorable legislation and to defeat poor legislation. Indifference, which tends to create bitter complaints, should never be one of the traits of the dental hygienist.

A deep concern for dentistry, dental hygiene and public service will assist the dental hygienist to achieve excellence in all areas of clinical performance, education and morality. How long after graduation does the dental hygienist's commitment last? Commitment to dental hygiene, in one way or another, is for a lifetime. Dental hygienists, by their very nature, are inquisitive and creative and search eagerly for new frontiers.

To achieve the goal of an idea is to face the hard actuality of choice and to conquer the hard necessity of decision. Knowledge, skills, attitudes, critical intelligence, energy, imagination and creativity are indispensable traits for the professional dental hygienist. Fulfillment of one's commitment requires that responsibilities be assumed with dedication, moral vitality and good judgment.

References

Motley, Wilma: Dental hygiene leadership. JADHA, 43:11-16, 1968.
Motley, Wilma: Message from the President. JADHA, 41:5-6, 1967.
Motley, Wilma: Message from the President. JADHA, 41:63-64, 1967.

Motley, Wilma: Message from the President. JADHA, 41:131-132, 1967.
Motley, Wilma: Message from the President. JADHA, 41:187-188, 1967.
Motley, Wilma: Message from the President. JADHA, 42:9-10, 1968.
Motley, Wilma: Message from the President. JADHA, 42:67-70, 1968.
Motley, Wilma: A dental hygienist's approach to modernization of dental hygiene laws. Presented to the Board Secretaries Conference, AADE, Chicago, September 1967.
Motley, Wilma: Message from the President. JADHA, 42:133-134, 1968.
Motley, Wilma: Message from the President. JADHA, 42:187-188, 1968.

Chapter 4

Jurisprudence

Definitions

Couvre-feu, or curfew, was a cover for controlling the fire. Medieval lights had to be put out at the ringing of an evening signal bell, and man, who lived in wooden houses, invented this metal cover so that he could secure his fire for the night. Applying the knowledge of dental jurisprudence can act as a *couvre-feu* for the professional person against legal action which might involve him or his associates. Avoiding lawsuits is far better than having all the help in the world to contest them. The use of common sense and tested principles can help safeguard the personal future of the dental hygienist and perhaps that of the dentist employer.

The French word *providens* was shortened to *prudens*—whence prudent, seeing ahead—and French and English *prude,* which originally meant wise. The wisdom of the law, therefore, is crystallized in jurisprudence (L. jus, juris, law).* *Jurisprudence* means science or philosophy of law, medical jurisprudence, forensic medicine (L. jus, juris, law + prudentia, knowledge, foresight).†

The Assyrians collected, systemized and supplemented Babylonian culture. Ashurbanipal (669-626 B.C.) is credited with having the first systematic library, and its contents date back to approximately 2,800 B.C. Sargon the Sumerian was the first man to collect a large library which he

* Shipley, Joseph T.: *Dictionary of Word Origins.* Paterson, N.J., Littlefield, Adams and Co., 1961.
† *Macmillan's Modern Dictionary.* New York, The Macmillan Co., 1938.

housed at Nineveh. Research in these collections indicates that the Code of Hammurabi established the concept of civil and penal responsibility of the physician. It shows that the practice of medicine and dentistry was regulated as far back as 2,250 B.C. by the Babylonians. The professions had advanced far enough to warrant public esteem and to be rewarded with adequate fees, set according to rank or position of the patient and the difficulty of the case and prescribed and regulated by law. There were strict penalties, not death but perhaps the loss of a hand, for malpractice and for the unsuccessful outcome of surgical procedures. Drugs, administered by priests who consulted an extensive pharmacopoeia, were used in those years for "bloodless" medicine.

Forensic dentistry deals with the relationships between dentistry and the law. The international term *forensic odontology* is considered to be part of the broad field of forensic dentistry. It is concerned with identification of persons based on dental evidence and deals with the proper handling of this evidence and the evaluation and presentation of dental findings. *Dental jurisprudence* might be the term used to describe other aspects of forensic dentistry, including statutes regulating dental practice, professional liability, professional incorporation and other legal aspects of the practice of dentistry.*

In presenting this subject there are two alternatives: to state the law in correct and elaborate detail or to eliminate elements not pertaining directly to the issue at hand—in this case the dental hygienist. However, in performing the procedures associated with dental care, problems will be encountered that have legal implications; it is therefore necessary that both dentist and dental hygienist know laws affecting professional practice. Awareness of these laws may help avoid unpleasant litigation, but it does not replace the services of an attorney as needed.

Nature of Law

No definition of law is adequate for all purposes, for the law is flexible. It changes according to the interest or the type of problem presented. Frictions will always exist between people or groups of people, and laws are formulated to avoid as many frictions as possible by providing binding and enforceable rules of conduct. Some laws have been adapted from other countries, some were enacted because of individual needs of time and place, but most United States laws are based on English Common Law. Careful appraisal of laws shows that they give clues to social problems, ethics and development of the period during which they were adopted.

Originally it was the Headman who ruled the tribe and made judgments; judgments usually were followed by the next leader. Changing needs made

* Vale, Gerald L.: The dentist's expanding responsibilities: Forensic odontology. J. So. Calif. Dent. Assoc., 37:248, 1969.

alterations necessary so laws would remain effective and relevant to contemporary situations. An outstanding characteristic of common or unwritten law is its flexibility because it provides principles which can be applied to hundreds of cases. Written laws are also used in conjunction with common law.

Roman law, which was very detailed, tried to cover all situations. By outlining a large variety of circumstances, the Roman law provided the judges with a basis for determining the issue. Europeans adopted this type of civil law or code. Some of our states, because of ethnic origin of early colonizers, have adopted or followed French or Spanish codes; other states have adapted common law in an effort to clarify and simplify the law. In spite of all attempts to make the law clear and understandable, attorneys and judges are still needed to interpret, to explain and to apply the law to a given case.

The principle of *stare decisis* (stand by the decided cases) means that principles once accepted should generally survive. Future actions can then depend on the stability of the law. Laws, however, can be changed when it becomes evident that there is public dissatisfaction or when judges overrule a decision, thus changing policy to meet current demands. The Constitution and Acts of Congress are the supreme law of the land, yet each state is sovereign in many respects. Among these is the right of each state to form its own requirements for qualification to practice dentistry and dental hygiene, the time within which a suit may be brought, and variances in interpretation of negligence. Because of these sovereign rights, no rule necessarily applies in all states. Law is a complex subject which has been divided into groups with further subdivisions. No attorney can keep all this information in mind but must be able to research and interpret it in a manner acceptable to the court.

Included within the professional responsibilities of the dentist is his need to apply legal rules governing business relationships so the business aspects of dental practice may be properly organized and supervised. There is need for knowledge of contracts for these are used in professional associations with another dentist, for financing purchases and for office leases. Outside the professional office it is advantageous to understand contracts to purchase or lease a home or income property.

It is no longer possible to practice a profession without relying on other professions. A suit involving personal injury would require an attorney to consult a physician or dentist regarding the nature, extent and prognosis of the injury so that the case can be presented properly; the dentist would not go to court without being represented by an attorney. The dentist, and quite possibly the dental hygienist, can be in court either as a plaintiff or a defendant, or may be called as a witness, either ordinary or expert. In dental practice there are standards of care to be observed and practitioners must be familiar with all aspects of these standards.

Types of Law

It is important for the dentist and the dental hygienist to have some understanding of the law as it pertains to contracts and torts. Technically contracts are "express" (specific agreement, either verbal or written, between the parties) or "implied" (no agreement—a contract is created solely by operation of law). An express contract involves mutual obligation (promises by each party) and consideration (something of value).

A tort is a civil wrong independent of contract. A tort (in law) deals with a private wrong done to a person or property for which a civil (not criminal) action can be brought and for which compensation can be claimed. Torts include: trespass, damage to property, seduction, invasion of privacy, slander, libel, intentional injury by assault and battery, negligent performance or failure to perform the duties of the patient-doctor (dental hygienist) relationship, and harm intentionally inflicted by the dentist (dental hygienist) upon the patient.

Torts are classified in two main subdivisions: intentional and negligent. Intentional torts are acts which are intentional; thus, the defendant is responsible for the results even if there are no actual damages. Trespass is one example. The dentist who slaps a child patient to secure cooperation in dental treatment has committed the intentional tort of battery (battery requires a touching, assault a threatened touching). Technical assault is the unconsented touching of the patient, i.e. the removal of a tooth without consent.

Malpractice is a subdivision of negligent torts. Liability is the concept which allows a person to collect a malpractice judgment from his dentist or dental hygienist or from the insurance carrier and, in other situations, which makes one person responsible for damage to another person or to property. Insurance which pays for such judgments is known as liability insurance and most such policies contain subdivisions of bodily injury liability and property damage liability.

A third type of legal actions are criminal cases. A crime is an act which is punishable by the state by fine, imprisonment, or death. A person can be guilty of both a crime and a tort and be liable to punishment by the state and an assessment for civil damages. This category includes acts ranging from parking violations through grand larceny to murder.

Malpractice in dentistry and dental hygiene can be defined in terms of acts of commission and acts of omission—failing to perform an act that a reasonable and prudent man would perform, or performing one which a reasonable and prudent man would not perform. Either case, performance or non-performance, must result in injury to the plaintiff before a lawsuit can be instituted. Malpractice, then, is simply professional negligence.

The law says that negligence is the failure to use due care, or the lack of due care, and it is the jury who determines whether or not the conduct met the required standards. The jury may believe one witness and not another; while the verdict of the jury usually stands, the judge may reduce the amount of damages awarded. The jury usually reflects the community's concept of the standards of care which should be expected of the professional person.

The State Board of Dental Examiners take some disciplinary actions for it supervises and administers established rules and regulations and their violation by dentists, dental hygienists, dental assistants and dental laboratory technicians.

Steps of Legal Action

The purpose of a lawsuit is to secure and enforce civil rights. First the facts of the case must be collected and the proper application of legal rules determined. Trial may be by jury or before a judge but, because of the complexity of laws and because the average individual is totally unfamiliar with court procedures, a qualified attorney should be in charge.

Witnesses and evidence may be requested or produced. A jury will be called, questioned and accepted or rejected. To assist jurors, counsel for each side outlines the case and what each counselor intends to prove. According to rules of the court on admissible and inadmissible evidence, questioning and cross-examination of the plaintiff then follow. If there has been an error in trial, the attorney may move for a new trial, and if this is granted, the whole procedure is reenacted. Otherwise final judgment is subject to review only by an appellate court.

The issues of accepted standards of care, the period and extent of disability, the act that was the basis for complaint, and cause of damages which followed all require expert witness testimony. "Did the instrument break?" "Was a fragment of the root left?" are questions of fact which may require radiographic interpretation by an expert witness; pain and suffering experienced and the cost of treatment may also need such testimony.

Problems of Practice

If the dentist chooses to be an employee of another dentist, he is relieved of the responsibilities of conducting an office, but this employment does not eliminate all of his liability. In private practice or in federal military service he may be held solely liable for acts of malpractice, or jointly with his employer. As an alternative, the dentist may choose to become an associate of an established dental practitioner. Here, too, someone else shares in responsibilities of the office, either equally or in relationship of employer-employee, but liability for acts of malpractice is still the responsibility of the individual.

Federal and state governments require employers to withhold taxes such as social security and income tax, plus contribute to certain employee benefits, and to pay into workmen's compensation insurance funds. Failure to withhold government taxes results in penalties, and failure to provide workmen's compensation insurance can result in criminal penalties, including fine and imprisonment. The uninsured employer is personally liable for medical bills and lifetime disability benefits to his employees who are injured on the job, and such a debt is not dischargeable in bankruptcy, and is a lien on all present and future assets of the employer.

Dentists in practice face other problems. *Respondeat superior,* a rule of the laws of agency, makes the employer responsible for injuries caused by employees in carrying out instructions of the employer. For instance, if the dentist requests his dental assistant to go to the dental supply house for him, and while driving on the errand she negligently collides with another car, causing damage, the dentist will be held responsible. Dental patients are "business invitees" and the person who treats them, whether he is an employer or an employee, is responsible for their safety on the premises and therefore is liable for any injuries suffered by the patient. Potential or confirmed drug addicts can create problems in the office as well as with the Bureau of Narcotic Enforcement. Water overflowing and fire from open flames are common causes of damage not only to the primary office but to premises of other tenants for which the dentist may be held responsible.

Duties of the Doctor to the Patient

Possession of a license does not mean that the dentist must accept or treat any person as a patient. Refusal may be based on any reason except the patient's race, creed or color. The dentist may be too busy, the case may be gratuitous or the patient may be personally unacceptable. Only when the patient has been accepted does the law impose duties upon both the dentist and the patient.

Implied conditions for the dentist are that he is licensed, that he use reasonable care and skill, standard drugs, materials and techniques, that he complete the work in a reasonable length of time, that he will not dismiss or abandon the patient without giving him the opportunity to secure other services, and that his fees will be reasonable.

Once the relationship is begun, both the dentist and patient can consider that it will continue until the work is completed; the relationship, however, may be terminated by mutual consent or withdrawal of either party. Without a written contract this termination may be for personal reasons, inability to secure results, termination of practice or an extended absence from practice. Notification of such termination must be in writing and care must continue a reasonable length of time in order to allow the patient to secure another dentist's services. Single services started must be finished; for example, a prepared cavity must be filled before service is terminated. If the dentist goes away on an extended vacation, provision must be made for treatment of emergencies of patients under treatment, and the patient should be alerted to this procedure.

Instructions to the patient must be reasonable, and be given in a manner he can understand. This is important, for a legal decision might be based on whether or not the dentist gave explicit and clear instructions. The burden of proof lies mainly with the plaintiff to prove damage, negligence or breach of contract. Information concerning the patient's health must not be disclosed except in court, and then only if the patient agrees, for this is a privileged communication. Such information is given only to help the dentist correctly diagnose and treat the patient.

Duties of the Patient to the Doctor

The patient is legally required to pay a reasonable and agreed fee for services rendered, to cooperate and to follow instructions. Reasonable fees usually are not questioned, and any fee expressly agreed to before the work is begun cannot be questioned even if it is above the usual fee for such service. The method of payment may be by a definite understanding at a specified time for each service rendered, or by regular payments. The person responsible for payment of dental fees should be apprised of services being rendered. Ordinarily, husbands are liable for work done for wives, fathers for children. Since a guardian is not always responsible for bills incurred, this should be clarified before proceeding with treatment.

It is incumbent on the patient to cooperate and follow instructions given him. If a product's brand name is given for use in a specific treatment, and the patient substitutes another product which does not produce the desired results, the patient is held to be at fault. It is important, however, that explicit and clear directions be given by the dentist, for the decision can be based on this point.

Malpractice

When a person professes some special knowledge or skill and offers a service to society, those who accept the service assume that they will be given ordinary and diligent care. If the practitioner shows neglect leading to injury, the courts are expected to support a claim against him. In legal parlance this is the principle of "due care." Due care includes sincerity, attentiveness, a willingness to learn from experience and to profit by previous mistakes. Due care also implies moral earnestness and intelligence.

The effect of this doctrine on the practice of dentistry requires that if the dentist knows, or as a reasonable man should have "known," of hazards inherent in his treatment, he is under a legal obligation to inform his patients of these hazards prior to commencing treatment. The law takes the position that you *do* know what you *should* know. This is a convincing argument for the professional to keep abreast of current knowledge of dentistry. Today's techniques and drugs may be outmoded in just a few years. To continue to use outmoded techniques and drugs with resultant injury is malpractice. You cannot warn your patient of side effects and hazards if you do not know what they are.

Proof of good practice is essential in order to win a dental malpractice lawsuit and the most acceptable evidence is adequate written records. The rules of evidence used in the United States will permit any and all dental records to be admitted into evidence as exceptions to the hearsay rule. The jury can take these records into the room where they will make their decision; therefore, if the records are complete, accurate and legible they can be a great help in proving innocence.

The minimum essential elements to prove good practice are an adequate, signed, dated, patient health history; an adequate and informed consent; adequate radiographs. If general anesthesia, intravenous sedation, or analgesia is to be used, even more elements are necessary: an adequate ambulatory anesthesia record; an adequately equipped office, including resuscitative devices; qualified personnel.

The first essential element of good practice, written records, is the adequate, signed and dated patient health history. Every physician and dentist is required to inform himself as fully as possible of the patient's physical condition. The patient is under no obligation to describe medical problems unless asked; if he suffers injury due to lack of provable knowledge of prior medical history, the doctor will be held strictly accountable. If the dentist is in doubt of any condition identified in the health history, the patient's physician should be consulted. A patient may deliberately or accidentally misinform the dentist about his state of health, but if the health history is signed by the patient it can be proven that an attempt was made to secure accurate information. The health history is reviewed periodically, for the professional operator is required to remain aware of the patient's health and any changes subsequent to initial questioning.

The heading of the health history should include name, address, telephone number, sex, date of birth, marital status, height and weight. The patient should be required to write "yes" or "no" rather than check or circle questions so that he cannot accuse someone else of having filled in wrong answers. Specific questions should be asked, the type and number depending on the kind of dental practice. The history should close with the date and the patient's signature, or if the patient is a minor the signature of the parent or guardian.

Questions might include:

Yes or No

1. Is your general health good? _____

2. Has there been any change in your general health in the last year? _____

3. My last physical examination was on _____

4. Were the results normal? _____

Yes or No

5. My physician's name and address are: _____

_____

6. Are you now under the care of physician? _____

7. If yes, who? _____

8. What condition is being treated? _____

9. Do you need or are you planning to have any surgery? _____

10. What is your blood type? _____ Have you ever had a transfusion?_____

11. Have you ever had a serious illness or operation? _____

12. If yes, what? _____

Do you wear a pacemaker? _____

13. Have you been hospitalized in the last five years? _____

14. If yes, what was the problem? _____

15. Do you have any of the following diseases or problems? _____

Anemia _____ Allergies: Food _____ Drug _____

Which foods? _____ Drugs _____

Arthritis or rheumatism _____

Asthma _____ Other respiratory difficulties _____
(sinus, emphysema, hay fever)

Cardiovascular disease; arteriosclerosis _____

coronary insufficiency _____ coronary occlusion _____

high _____ low _____ blood pressure

Diabetes _____

Fainting spells _____ dizziness _____ convulsions _____ epilepsy _____

Hepatitis _____ jaundice _____ liver disease _____

Nephritis _____ kidney trouble _____

Rheumatic heart disease _____ Gastrointestinal ulcers _____

Tuberculosis _____ persistent cough _____ cough blood _____

16. Are you taking any of the following?

Antibiotics: Penicillin _____ Mycin _____ Sulfa _____

Anticoagulants _____

Aspirin _____ Anacin _____ Other pain or headache pill _____

Cortisone _____ Digitalis _____ Other drug for heart _____

Insulin _____ Orinase _____ Similar drug _____

Medicine for high blood pressure _____

Tranquilizers _____

Yes or No

17. Do you bleed excessively following a cut, surgery or wound? _____

    If yes, are you a hemophiliac? _____ Other reason _____

18. Have you ever had surgery or x-ray treatment of a tumor, growth
    or other condition of your mouth or lips? _____

19. Have you ever had a local or general anesthetic? _____

20. Have you ever had an unfavorable reaction or result from local
    or general anesthesia? _____ If yes, what? _____

21. Have you experienced any unfavorable reaction or result from
    previous dental treatment? _____ If yes, what? _____

22. Have you ever had any other disease, condition or problem not
    listed that I should know about? _____ If yes, what? _____

23. (For women) Are you pregnant? _____

    Do you have menstrual problems? _____

Date _____ Signature _____

Blood pressure _____ Pulse _____ Temperature _____

Doctor's notes

No one should utilize all of the foregoing questions. They merely illustrate the number and type of questions which can be asked. A satisfactory health history should be worked out for the particular type of practice. For example, an oral surgeon would certainly want to add questions such as "Have you had anything to eat or drink in the last four hours?" and "Is there someone to drive you home?"

The second essential element to prove good dental practice is the adequate and signed informed consent. If the dentist cannot prove that the patient consented to the dentistry he is guilty of technical assault. Since 1960 the courts have required that the patient be informed in advance of any adverse effects of the dentistry. This doctrine of informed consent places a heavy, and from a practical standpoint impossible, standard on physicians and dentists. To warn each patient of all the possible hazards of treatment could result in deterring the patient from necessary care. But, if the dentist can reasonably foresee severe problems, then he must warn the patient in advance of these hazards and give the patient the right to determine whether or not he wishes to assume the risk and proceed. The problem then is one of proof. The patient may deny that he gave an informed consent because there was in fact no warning; or he forgot or did not hear or understand the warning due to his general apprehension at the moment; or the dentist made light of the hazards and did not impress the patient with their importance; or the patient is lying in order to recover damages.

Implied, verbal and written consents are common in the everyday practice of dentistry. By implication of law, the patient, by the act of coming to the dental office, agrees to (probably) oral prophylaxis, radiographs and diagnosis. If he states his dental problem and asks for care, consent is implied. Implied consent extends no further but will prevent a technical assault on the above grounds and will permit collection of a reasonable fee. It is good policy to dismiss the patient if he will not consent to radiographs, and *in no case do anything forbidden by him.* If the patient refuses to have radiographs made, other work should not be done.

Almost all dental service is provided on the basis of a verbal agreement. Such consents are perfectly valid legally; the problem is one of proof. If the lower left second molar is extracted and the patient later claims that he consented to extraction of the lower left first molar, only the jury can determine the actual scope of the consent. If the consent was in writing, the patient cannot deny it, so common sense, good practice and the law dictate that written consents be obtained for all important dentistry.

General consents to "any and all dental services to be rendered by . . ." are of little or no help since it is impossible to determine just what the parties did agree to. The court will throw out such evidence on the basis that it was too vague and indefinite.

There is no such thing as "a consent form" for all dental situations and all types of dental practice. It should be a written summary of the treatment to which the dentist and the patient have agreed, dated and signed by the patient. This will avoid problems in fee collections and difficulties in defense of claims for malpractice or technical assault. A short statement will sometimes suffice but, in more complicated dentistry, the consent should be a part of the written treatment plan. It should cover the possibility of extending the surgery provided that the extension is a corollary to the original plan. An authorization to use any anesthetic deemed proper in the opinion of the dentist should be included, as should a specific acknowledgment by the patient that he has been warned of known possible hazards involved in the treatment.

Who may sign the consent? Adults may sign for themselves or for their minor children, or as guardians of minors. Each state has its own rules on minority, defining it in terms of age, marital status, or sex.

If it is possible, consent should be obtained from both parents of a minor. Usually if the parents are separated, the mother has custody and her consent would avoid technical assault charges, but the father, who pays the bill, might refuse unless he signed the consent. If the parents are not available to sign a consent, verbal consent may be obtained by telephone, but the dental assistant should be on a second telephone, and both dentist and assistant should initial the entry recording the verbal consent. If the parents cannot be reached, treatment should be delayed until their return unless it is a life-endangering emergency.

An emergency is usually defined as the immediate danger of death or serious bodily harm when the patient is unable to give consent because he is unconscious or out of his senses. If the patient is a child and the parents cannot be reached, implied consent is presumed in an emergency, or the patient can be referred to the county hospital.

It is difficult to know what to do for a minor entirely on his own. If he lies to you he is forgiven for he is a minor and the parents might claim technical assault, or he may legally not pay if he disaffirms the contract for non-necessaries.

Another cardinal rule for consents and health histories is not to rely on the first one taken. Health information should be updated continually to reflect the patient's physical changes. The same is true for consents. Always secure the patient's consent to any new treatment, for it is unsafe to assume that because he consents once he will consent again.

Many everyday routine dental office procedures can become bases for malpractice suits if due care and good judgment are not exercised by all dental personnel involved. Lack of accepted techniques of sterilization of hypodermic needles or instruments can cause or spread infection in the patient or between patients. Root tips broken off or pushed into the maxillary sinus cavity and delayed postoperative treatments are hazards of oral surgery. Foreign bodies aspirated because of lack of use of rubber dam, a slip of the bur or disk which cuts into soft tissue and extensive drug burns can also be causes for patient action against the professional person. Ordinarily the statute of limitations begins when the act is committed, not when the damage is discovered. The time limitation on a breach of contract is usually longer than that on tort actions for personal injuries.

Liability for Acts of Others

"The master is liable for the acts of his servant" and "the principal is liable for the acts of his agent" are phrases which apply to the dentist and his liability for the acts of others.

In the dentist-patient relationship, the dentist acts as an independent agent since he performs a special service for the patient, doing the work in his own way, and for a fee. If he cannot do the work alone he hires someone, whom he directs, to assist him. This is known as a "master-servant" relationship. The master then may be held liable for the acts of the servant which cause damage. When an assistant is given authority to enter into business arrangements on behalf of the employer this relationship becomes that of "principal and agent."

To determine the liability of the employer for the act of another it is necessary to first determine whether the servant or agent relationship existed at the time the act took place. Even though the dentist may be present, it is possible for an assistant to injure the patient by burning him with hot water or modeling compound or electrical equipment, by handing the dentist the wrong solution, by allowing infection through abrasion from an instrument.

Dental Hygienists

Although the scope of the dental hygienist's practice is limited, the high standards of care and skill which the profession of dental hygiene expects of its members require the demonstration of excellence in all areas. The failure to provide care and skill, or the act of negligence, is known as malpractice.

All state dental practice acts require that the dental hygienist work under the supervision or direction of a licensed dentist. Some states interpret this in a very strict manner, inserting "direct" before the word supervision or direction, meaning that the employing dentist must be in the office while the dental hygienist is working. Other states interpret supervision or direction as meaning that the employing dentist must be present in the office a majority of the time while the dental hygienist is working. The dental hygienist could be faced with unanticipated emergencies or unusual circumstances requiring assistance; therefore, it is unwise for the dental hygienist to work when the dentist is not present.

An Employee

By law, the dental hygienist, working under the supervision or direction of a licensed dentist, paid either by salary or by commission, or a combination of these two methods, whether or not the patient pays for the service rendered, is considered an employee, not a separate contractor or self-employed.

The following is a copy of Internal Revenue Rule #58-268, pages 353-354.

> For Federal employment tax purposes, a dental hygienist is an employee of the dentist for whom she performs services, where she reports to the dentist's office on designated days of each week and gives oral prophylaxis to the patients of the dentist under an agreement with the dentist providing for the payment of a fee of a specified percentage of the amount charged each patient treated, whether or not collected from the patient.
>
> Advice has been requested as to the status, for Federal employment tax purposes, of a dental hygienist who gives oral prophylaxis treatment to the patients of a dentist under the circumstances described below.
>
> A practicing dentist has engaged the services of a licensed dental hygienist to give oral prophylaxis treatments to his patients in his office. The treatment consists of removing calcified deposits and cleaning teeth. The dental hygienist performs her services on one or two days of each week under an oral agreement which provides that she shall receive a percentage of the amount charged the patient for each treatment. Such fee is paid whether or not collected from the patient. The dental hygienist is qualified to render services without instructions from the dentist and uses discretion with respect to the methods employed in the services. She does not solicit or secure patients but does arrange the time the patient shall return for any subsequent treatments required. She also charts on each patient's card the location of any suspected carious lesions as well as any deviations from the normal observed in the course of treatment. She holds herself available to perform oral prophylaxis ser-

vices for the dentist on days selected to suit the convenience of both parties. Her name does not appear on the office door of the dentist, on his business cards, in the building directory, or in the classified section of the telephone directory, and she does not advertise her services to the public. All office expenses are borne by the dentist and he provides office space for the hygienist and furnishes all necessary supplies and equipment. The services of the hygienist may be terminated by either party at any time. The hygienist performs similar services for other dentists on days that she does not report to the office of the dentist herein concerned.

Under section 3121(d)(2) of Federal Insurance Contributions Act (chapter 21, subtitle C, Internal Revenue Code of 1954), the term "employee" means any individual who, under the usual common law rules applicable in determining the employer-employee relationship has the status of an employee. The guides for determining, under such rules, whether an employer-employee relationship exists are found in section 31.3121 (d)-1(c) of the Employment Tax Regulations. Whether an individual is an employee or an independent contractor is largely a question of fact to be determined from the circumstances of a particular case.

Upon the basis of the information presented, it is concluded that the dentist exercises or has the right to exercise such control and direction over the dental hygienist in the performance of her services as is necessary, under the usual common law rules to establish the relationship of employer and employee. Accordingly, it is held that the hygienist is an employee of the dentist for the purposes of the taxes imposed under the Federal Insurance Contributions Act.

The foregoing conclusion also applies for purposes of the Federal Unemployment Tax Act and the Collection of Income Tax at Source on Wages.*

It is clear from this ruling that the dentist employer must follow accepted accounting procedures, make the proper tax deductions from each pay check and make payments to the Internal Revenue Service of the withheld taxes along with the employer's contribution to the employee's Social Security account. The dental hygienist is obligated to report all earnings and to pay any remaining tax due, or if indicated can request a refund of the overpayment of withholding tax. Failure to fulfill these tax obligations and those imposed by the individual states can result in the guilty parties being forced years later to pay not only the actual amount of the taxes previously due but accrued interest on that amount and any penalties imposed.

Many dentists are now establishing retirement plans for themselves and their employees under provision of the Keough Act.† As an employee, the dental hygienist who meets the eligibility requirements can participate in this benefit.

The Keough plan allows self-employed persons to set aside, on a tax deferred basis, 15% of their income up to $7,500 annually for investment in a qualified retirement plan. A corporate employee can set aside 100% of the average of the three highest years of earnings on a tax-deferred basis, not to exceed $75,000.

Dentists who use either of these plans must also provide similar pension programs for their employees on a nondiscriminatory basis. Qualified em-

* Internal Revenue Code of 1954: Chapters 23 and 24, Subtitle C. Also Sections 3306, 3401; 31.3306 (i)-1. And also compare Rev. Rul. 57-380, C.B. 1957-2, 634, and Rev. Rul. 57-381, C.B. 1957-2, 636.

† Internal Revenue Code: Retirement Plans for Self-Employed Individuals, Reaffirmed, 1974.

ployees include those 25 years of age or older who have been employed full time for at least three years. Other changes in the law allow up to $750 to be sheltered regardless of the percentage limitations and payment may now be made up to the date for filing the tax return. Except in case of death or permanent disability benefits may not be withdrawn before age 59½ and must begin by age 70½ without payment of stiff penalties which are meant to discourage premature withdrawal.

Depending on the plan chosen by the dentist he must contribute an amount equal to 15% of each employee's income to a pension plan, or establish a retirement program that would pay retirement income equal to the three highest years of the employee's earnings.

Employees of a non-profit tax exempt foundation or corporation organized for charitable, religious, scientific, or educational purposes, or any public school system or university may be eligible for a tax-sheltered annuity for their retirement. A tax accountant or attorney should be consulted for details of qualifications.

Additionally, for the first time, employees not covered by a pension plan can establish an Individual Retirement Account. The annual deduction limits are the lesser of 15% of income or $1,500. Married couples can compute deductions separately providing both qualify. Investment options and withdrawal formula are essentially the same as for other Keough plans. IRS publications are available.

Some dental hygienists and their employers would prefer that the classification be that of independent contractor rather than employee, thus eliminating the extra bookkeeping of tax accounting and allowing certain other deductions on the yearly income tax return. If the dental hygienist were to be classified as an independent contractor and worked for a percentage of the fee charged the patient, the dentist then could become guilty of "fee splitting," a practice prohibited by law. When all the advantages and disadvantages of being an employee or an independent contractor are weighed, more often than not the hygienist profits by being declared an employee.

Liability

Responsibility for personal errors is incumbent on the individual. Although the law of agency prevails in this situation, which means that the dentist can be sued for the employee's misdeed, suit can be instituted against the responsible individual. No professional liability insurance carried by the dentist protects the dental hygienist unless that individual's name is specified in the policy or in a rider attached to the policy. If a suit is instituted against the dental hygienist, or dental hygienist and the dentist jointly, the dentist's professional liability insurance company might or might not provide legal defense or pay judgments for the accused dental hygienist. There is no contractual requirement to do so unless the dental hygienist is named in the liability policy. If the insurance company did defend the dental hygienist and a judgment was rendered against the defendant, the insuring company could demand reimbursement. A personal policy carried by the dental hygienist will offer protection in such a situation. As with the supervising dentist and the employee dental hygienist, the policy protecting the dental hygienist who works in a supervisory capacity does not cover those persons being supervised.

An increase in responsibility accompanies the growth of professional stature. The dental hygienist, therefore, becomes liable legally and financially for injury or loss to another due to error or omission during professional activities. It is possible for a single lawsuit to result not only in a judgment for a large sum of money but in time spent in court, diminished earning power, pain and suffering.

A comprehensive liability insurance program should include personal liability, premises liability and professional liability, with the best protection secured by carrying these in one company. There can be a question as to which type of liability the case will be tried under, and if one company is handling it all there can be no dispute between companies about the defense. Juries determine questions of fact; judges determine questions of law. The court decides whether personal or professional negligence is involved.

Patients can claim that they were injured during the performance of professional duties or that there was failure to provide the care expected of a competent dental hygienist. A patient may slip on a wet sidewalk, fall because of a hole in the sidewalk or because of some obscure obstruction, or slip on an over-waxed floor and bring suit for damages suffered. The dental hygienist can also be liable for damages suffered by persons accompanying the patient as well as by the patient himself. For example, the child who accompanies his mother on an office visit climbs on a stool and falls, injuring himself, or cuts himself on instruments, or burns himself with chemicals which he may reach. These injuries can happen while the operator is present and caring for the patient, but children should never be left alone in the reception room or an operatory whether they are patients or are accompanying the patient.

Safeguards and Insurance

Prevention is the best defense against malpractice. Money is only a part of insurance; safety measures put into effect are also good insurance. An efficient, sanitary office is a good beginning. Each patient should receive meticulous attention to all the requirements of good dental hygiene practice, which include limiting practice to fields within the qualifications of the operator, knowing legal duty to the patient and practicing safety measures.

Ideal records which would be presentable in court will clearly and legibly show the date and services rendered for each patient and will be complete enough to indicate that nothing was neglected. All charts, diagnoses, radiographs, carbon copies of laboratory specifications and prescriptions, and correspondence to or about the patient should be filed in the record folder. In this way proof of the patient's condition and treatment can be produced at once. If the patient discontinues treatment, records should indicate this decision. It is wise to write the patient, with a copy for the file, advising him against this course and informing him of the need to continue treatment with another dentist.

An adequate health history is a requisite part of diagnosis. No dental hygienist should treat a patient without a complete health history which is current or at least has been reviewed to be certain there have been no adverse changes in the patient's health. Established office policy dictates whether this will be a minimum health history or very extensive. If there is any question about the patient's physical condition and ability to accept treatment, the dentist or physician should be consulted. Dentists are now being encouraged to take the patient's blood pressure and to inquire about a pacemaker. The patient who wears a pacemaker requires special attention while in the dental office. In addition to being aware of the potential hazards to the patient, office personnel should know the procedures to follow if the pacemaker should be shut off accidentally. A minimum health history should contain information outlined on page 61.

After the health history form has been completed by the patient, careful, thorough charting of all existing conditions in the new patient's mouth is one of the more important records to be made. In addition to recording facts shown by a visual examination, periodontal pocket depth should be explored and complete oral radiographic surveys should be secured. When this information is available the dentist can make a comprehensive diagnosis with assurance that nothing affecting the patient's oral health is being overlooked or neglected. Defects and anomalies can be discovered and corrected or referred for special care.

Violent deaths in the United States are steadily increasing and positive identifications are often necessary for adjustment of insurance claims, estate settlement, remarriage or criminal prosecution. Visual examination, fingerprints and personal effects are used as means of identification but cannot always be reliable. Although teeth are highly susceptible to disease in life, they, and their restorations, are the least destructible parts of the body after death. There are so many individual characteristics of each mouth that it is unlikely that any two would be alike. Thus forensic odontology is a reliable science. Age up to fifteen years can be ascertained by complete oral radiographs, with panoramic radiographs the most useful type for identification.

Throughout the years teeth have been used as identification for a wide variety of reasons. About 66 A.D., so historians tell us, Nero's mistress, Sabina, demanded the head of his wife on a silver platter. To be sure that there had not been a substitution, Sabina made positive identification by means of a black anterior tooth which the luckless wife was known to have. General Joseph Warren, the physician who sent Paul Revere on his famous ride, was buried after the Battle of Bunker Hill in an unmarked grave. At the end of the Revolutionary War, Revere, dentist-silversmith, identified the body by the silver and ivory bridge which he had fabricated for General Warren. And Adolf Hitler's charred body was at least tentatively identified by his teeth which had survived the fire. Bite marks are also used in criminal cases for identification of the assailant.

Identification by a family member or friend can be mistaken through human error in judgment or through the emotional stress of the moment. Mistaken identity can also be willful in order to hide facts, but identification through teeth usually is reliable. These facts make it imperative to chart carefully each patient's existing restorations, missing teeth and removable appliances. Many dentists chart only the work they do. Their records actually are incomplete. Some of the more unique information about the patient's mouth, such as abnormalities and impactions, should be recorded, too, as these are even more positive means of identification. If photography is possible, intra-oral photographs should be obtained as an additional record. Color photographs showing silver or gold restorations are best.

As a diagnostic aid as well as a legal safeguard, complete oral radiographic surveys are essential for a new patient, and should be made on a stated routine basis thereafter. It is particularly necessary for children to have a radiographic survey in order to detect missing or supernumerary teeth, early carious lesions, and the relationships of head, jaw and teeth for orthodontic evaluation. Adults need oral diagnostic radiographs regularly for detection of dental caries, abscessed or impacted teeth, periodontal bone loss and other non-normal conditions.

The complete oral radiographic survey is a part of the doctor's records necessary to the comprehensive diagnosis. To avoid the possibility of the patient claiming ownership, wording of fee statements is critical. The patient who is billed for "X-rays" might have a chance of his ownership being upheld. Billing for "professional services" or "radiographic examination" is a safer procedure.

As another safeguard against legal involvements, instruments must be sterilized carefully, and equipment which cannot be sterilized must be sanitized. There are no shortcuts in sterilizing instruments. This is a procedure which requires meticulous attention to detail. The patient who sees evidence of this care as well as the rituals of handwashing and filling the drinking cup is reassured that his well-being is a paramount concern of the office. All instruments and equipment should be checked regularly to be sure that they are in good working condition, clean and sterile. Modern disposable dental items such as bracket table covers, headrest covers and patient towels make it far easier to maintain the chain of sterility.

Always check medication and dosage before handing prescription or medicament to the patient and never make substitutions without the dentist's knowledge and permission. Medicine should never be given in an unmarked container, and should be handed to an adult, never to a child. Be sure that dated supplies are up to date and that cupboards and drawers are clean. Never let the patient help himself from office supplies.

Assault, slander and libel are causes for legal action against the dental hygienist. Assault was defined earlier in this chapter as a threatened touching, technical assault the unconsented touching of the patient. Slander is oral defamation of character; libel is written defamation. Discretion is a necessary safety precaution required of this dental auxiliary. Many times it is difficult to be tactful, but the work of another dentist or dental hygienist should not be criticized. It is difficult, if not impossible, to know the circumstances under which the work was done, or even that the patient is reporting correctly. Fees of other offices, disclosure of confidences, or talk about any patient who could be identifiable are not proper or safe topics for discussion by the dental hygienist.

Any injury or damage to the patient which occurs with any possibility of charges being filed should be reported immediately to the insurance carrier by telephone, followed by a written report of the incident. It is never wise to inform the patient that liability insurance is carried, and no statement, either oral or written, should be made to him about liability for an act until the insurance company or an attorney has been consulted. Either one of these agencies is more experienced in legal actions than the dentist or dental hygienist and will be prepared to counsel the potential defendant.

What happens to the dental hygienist who follows the dentist-employer's orders to perform procedures not legalized in that state—removing crowns and fillings, injecting anesthetics or antibiotics, or taking study model impressions? If such illegal procedures are reported to the proper authorities, the dentist and the dental hygienist are subject to disciplinary action by the State Board of Dental Examiners, which will apply whatever penalties are stipulated in that state's dental practice act. Even though many schools are lawfully teaching these techniques related to the expansion of duties of the dental hygienist, in many states there is presently no legal basis for their performance in private practice. If the dental hygienist performs an illegal dental procedure which causes injury to the patient and results in a lawsuit, malpractice insurance is not applicable. The dental hygienist who illegally assumes these or other functions outside the purview of dental hygiene practice, whether at the request of the employer or by personal intent, is not only violating the law but is also violating personal and professional ethics.

Approximately thirty-five states have revised their dental practice acts to legalize the use of expanded function auxiliaries. These practice acts which vary a great deal represent extreme permissiveness to strict limitation; some allowing only reversible procedures, others including irreversible procedures. Not all points of law have been spelled out but will be decided in courts, making thirty-five interpretations possible.

The dentist, in all cases, is legally responsible for his own acts and those of his auxiliaries to whom he delegates certain functions, and the employee also has legal liabilities. Legal action after injury to the patient during treatment by an auxiliary will result in definitive court opinions. Until that time the legal implication of the utilization of expanded function auxiliaries cannot be known.

Personal Federal Tax Deductions

There are some income tax deductions which almost guarantee an audit of the return. The Internal Revenue Service is often willing to compromise, but it can be an uncomfortable experience and records must be complete. Current prime issues include deduction of employment agency fees when no job resulted, maintenance and depreciation on a home, gifts to children, short term trusts, corporate trust and E-Bond gifts. It does not mean that these deductions should be passed by, but that the rest of the return must be in order. Deductions are questionable, but misrepresenting income is fraud. It is advisable to consult a tax attorney if there is any doubt.

The use of computers which can compare and contrast information with norms in your category has changed the odds on the possibility of a tax audit. One of the best ways to avoid income tax audit is to be average. There are many tables published each year which show average deductions for various income brackets, but if there is proof for higher deductions they should be taken. Large deductions for business trips are always suspect.

Continuing education requirements of states to meet licensure renewal or professional organization membership qualifications are sure to increase travel and thereby create new tax situations. Some deductions are fairly standard, but allowance of other items can depend on accurate records kept by the taxpayer and the individuality of the tax examiner.

It is essential to establish the professional benefit of the meeting attended. Travel, meals, hotel accommodations and tuition are deductible items, but not costs of entertainment, and verification of dates and expenses should be available. If the trip is divided between business and pleasure only the business expense is deductible. A tax accountant should be consulted for details before an extended trip is taken.

If an arithmetic or statutory unallowable error (such as forgetting the one percent or three percent medical limitations) is made, the bill is for the difference plus interest. No appeals are allowed. If the return is questioned it is returned to the tax district and assigned to a tax auditor who makes the final decision on audit.

Damage suffered from fires, storms, theft and other natural or man-made calamities are deductible although casualty losses are scrutinized carefully. To be deductible a casualty must be sudden, unexpected or unusual. To claim a personal loss all deductions must be itemized, claiming only the decrease in the fair market value of property. The first $100 of any casualty loss (each case, not each item) cannot be claimed and any reimbursement (insurance or disaster relief) must be subtracted. Business losses are deductible in full.

Records are important in making such claims. Such things as ownership of the property, value before and after the casualty, cost of repairs, and the amount of insurance received. A camera can provide irrefutable proof of loss or protect the security deposit on an apartment. An all-inclusive file can document the home, all buildings from all sides, and all rooms and their contents, adding major improvements and additions to the contents. Photographs in color are preferable, and all should be dated. This file, which should be kept in a fireproof container or off the premises, can also serve as an inventory for determination of insurance needed. If a casualty occurs another series of photographs should be taken to establish the loss.

Three years is an adequate time to keep some records but tax returns should be kept indefinitely as should cancelled checks for tax payments, house records, stock records, gifts or inheritance. If tax returns are accidentally lost or destroyed copies may be secured from the IRS; however, they routinely feed tax returns to the shredder after six years.

Federal Laws Affecting Retail Credit

It is not usual for the dental hygienist to be responsible for making financial arrangements with patients or for collection of delinquent accounts. It is well, however, to be aware of some of the basic legalities of these office functions. An understanding of the law is vital because the law is binding and this knowledge can facilitate better patient relations.

Laws to be familiar with include the Federal Trade Commission's Guides against Debt Collection Deception; the Federal Communications Commission's Public Notice on Use of Telephone for Debt Collection Purposes; the Truth-in-Lending provision, Regulation Z of the Consumer Protection Act of 1968 and the Fair Credit Reporting Act (Title V of the Consumer Protection Act of 1968). Penalties for not observing them are great and could result from federal or class action suits filed by the patient.

In using the telephone to collect a debt the FTC will not tolerate subterfuge; it is necessary to state who is calling and why. Any legal action resulting from deception would be against the dentist employer.

The FCC also deals with what can and cannot be done via telephone, specifically invasion of privacy. If consideration is used and the delinquent patient is called during regular office hours, and a pleasant telephone manner is used in discussion of past due accounts, the law will never be a problem nor would violation be in question. The penalty for violation of this law would be the loss of the right to have a telephone in the business office.

The Truth-in-Lending provision, Regulation Z of the Consumer Protection Act of 1968, deals with the collection of payments. When a patient's account is to be paid in more than four installments, Regulation Z requires that a written disclosure of all pertinent information be made, regardless of whether or not a finance charge is to be made. If the patient decides on his own to pay in installments, or whenever convenient, this is not applicable.

The purpose of the Fair Credit Reporting Act is to protect the consumer against unreasonable denial of credit; he must be given an explanation and an opportunity to answer. Data from a report made by a credit bureau, or similar agency, need not be revealed, but the name and address of the agency *must be given* even though the patient may not ask for the information. Rejection on other grounds, such as age or employment, not related to credit information, should be justified to the patient. A safeguard from future law suits is the use of a form letter which courteously informs the patient that credit has been denied because he does not meet requirements and which has blanks for inserting name and address of the supplier of the information. This particular law gives the consumer a chance to correct his credit record or to build a good record after he has had trouble.

Corporation or Government as Employer

The dental hygienist employed by a dental corporation is bound by the same legal responsibilities and restrictions as in any other type of dental practice. There is the same employer-employee relationship and the same tax liabilities to be observed.

The dental hygienist employed by the federal government also observes these legalities but practices under one exception. As long as dental hygiene services are performed on the government base the license held may be from any state, not necessarily the one of present residence.

References

Ber, Joel: Where the IRS Would Rather Fight Than Switch, Dental Management, Harcourt, Brace Jovanovich Publication, February 1974, p. 15.

Blair, Virginia: You and the Law, JADAA, August 1974, p. 19.

Carnahan, Charles Wendell: *The Dentist and the Law,* St. Louis, C. V. Mosby Co., 1955.

Geylin, Martin: Tax-Free Annuity? Anyone? Dental Management, Harcourt, Brace Jovanovich Publication, February 1974, p. 52.

Green, David: What's the DIF on Your Tax Return? ibid, p. 18.

Keeling, Daniel B.: Lectures on Dental Jurisprudence, School of Dentistry, University of Southern California, Los Angeles, California.

Miller, Sidney L.: *Legal Aspects of Dentistry,* New York, G. P. Putnam's Sons, 1970.

Sienkiewicz, Richard Jr.: How Long to Hang on to Those Tax Records? Dental Management, Harcourt, Brace Jovanovich Publication, February 1974, p. 63.

Trumbull, Nicholas R.: The Good News About the Bad News, ibid, p. 28.

Wolfson, Edward: Expanded Duty Auxiliary Activity has Legal Implications, Dental Student News, September-October 1974, p. 4.

Chapter 5

History of Oral Hygiene

The overwhelming need for dental care which we see every day might cause us to believe that concern for the health and care of the mouth and teeth is a relatively new concept in our culture. On the contrary, these concerns, in greater or lesser degree, have been present since man evolved. Chimpanzees have been observed using a straw as a toothpick, presumably to alleviate an uncomfortable feeling of food impacted between the teeth, and it is reasonable to imagine that Neanderthal man did the same thing with a thorn, quill or stick of some kind.

It is no wonder that the mouth and teeth have been of great interest to man through countless centuries, for these are the physiologic organs through which he ingests food and liquids necessary for growth, survival and gustatory pleasure. These organs are also important components of the system by which he carried on a great measure of his communications. In addition, teeth have been used by man at various times for prehension, locomotion, transport, tools and secondary sex "weapons."

The evolution of oral hygiene has been linked closely with the culture, medicine and art of diversified groups of people throughout the world. Ritual, superstition, mysticism, medical knowledge and quackery, art and handicraft, trade and industry have all played a role in shaping oral hygiene into what we believe and accept today. Advertising only reinforces the fact that opportunities for dental health education are unlimited and urgently needed. If we are to believe the many claims of manufacturers of dentifrices, mouthwashes and other dental aids, the American public is still in the dark ages looking for some magic potion or abracadabra to cure its ills without effort or delay.

A comprehensive history of oral hygiene from the beginning of time would include detailed descriptions of the various ways that people cleansed and preserved their teeth and the reasons for those practices—whether they were the result of superstitious beliefs, esthetics, or a true desire for oral and general health. Tracing the evolution of the toothbrush from a pointed stick to the device used today would be a portion of the story, and dentifrices, mouthwashes and other implements would have their own sections. All of these are closely related to dentistry and its growth as well as to the changing socio-political-religious development of man over the years. Volumes have been written on each aspect of oral hygiene. This chapter traces the dentally related highlights of the early years of man to the late 1800's when the profession of dental hygiene was first seriously considered by dental practitioners. It culminates with a more detailed history of the profession of dental hygiene.

From Prehistoric Times Through the Middle Ages

Studies of animal remains 250 million years old show evidence of traumatic injury of dental origin and specimens of 100 million years ago show not only injury but evidence of disease caused by bacterial invasion. Remains of a dinosaur of that age indicate that he suffered from dental caries. *Homo monsteriensis,* 100,000 years ago, had to contend with retained deciduous teeth, impacted teeth, fractures and rickets. By 10,000 B.C. Neolithic man in Europe practiced the knocking out of teeth, and by 5,000 B.C. he was performing surgery on the skull. Although man was able to attend to some of his dental needs he also depended on supernatural assistance. The earliest known deity associated with the healing arts was Ea, invoked by the Babylonians as the ancient enemy of the tooth worm.

Because primitive man feared the unfamiliar, he attributed occult powers to any unexplainable phenomenon. Thus he believed that babies born with teeth were a menace and that early tooth eruption meant early senility. He also believed that teeth had miraculous powers, both good and evil, so he used powdered teeth as medicaments for illnesses, tartar from the teeth to heal bone fractures, and carried teeth to ensure luck or health or protection against the evil eye. Many other odd conclusions grew from the appearance of the teeth and even as late as 1865 people in France believed that the shape and arrangement of the teeth were a valid means of judging character.

In addition to using a primitive toothpick, early man probably chewed fragrant wood to sweeten his breath and perhaps found that the softened, chewed end could be used advantageously as a brush to clean his teeth and provide sensual pleasure. Persian Parsees included such cleansing in their religious rites as did the Mohammedans who used their miswak. The miswak was a dental fiber pencil, often made of arak wood rich in sodium bicarbonate. After soaking in water for twenty-four hours it was pounded until the plant fibers unravelled to form a sort of brush, the unbeaten part of the stick serving as a handle. According to religious law, the front teeth were cleansed first, then the side teeth, always with prayers, for "A prayer preceded by the toothpick is worth seventy-five ordinary prayers." The use of these sticks spread from Arabia and Persia to India, China and Japan, where Buddhists cited the evils of not cleaning the teeth, then to Africa where chewsticks are still used. The people of Israel, too, were concerned with hygiene; Moses defined laws which showed appreciation for care of the teeth. The custom of keeping a splinter of wood or toothpick in the mouth all day some now feel was an early attempt at the practice of orthodontics.

We have every reason to believe that the teeth were an important concern to people of the Egyptian Empire period for the archeological evidence shows that they attempted not only to clean their teeth but to replace missing teeth and to ornament the teeth still in the mouth. The earliest known toilet set, consisting of toothpick, ear scoop and tweezers, was found in the Ningal Temple at Ur, dated in 3500 B.C.

The Papyrus of Ebers has a brief section on dentistry which deals with fractures of the jaw, injuries to the lips and chin and dislocation of the jaw, but does not mention fillings or prostheses. It is known that, of the many specialists in medicine, dentists were the physicians who specialized in treating and caring for the teeth. Egyptian symbols interpreted by archeologists show designations of treater or maker of teeth, i.e. Tooth Worker, the hieroglyphics being an eye and a tusk. The earliest known dentist, Hesi-Ré, Great One (Chief) of the Toothers and Physicians, was symbolized by a bird and a tusk. Egyptians of this early period apparently did not suffer extensively from dental caries; however, records show that despite the efforts of dentists Egyptians had "loose teeth," undoubtedly indicative of periodontal involvement. The ritual of the dead, written in great detail by the Babylonians as well as the Egyptians, included mouth opening and washing for purification so that the deceased could eat and speak in the hereafter. The small vials used by the Egyptians 2000-1785 B.C. in this ritual have been found by archeologists.

In widely separated parts of the known world dental care was one of the prime concerns of ancient civilizations. In Babylonia, Hammurabi wrote codes to protect the patient and to govern the practice of medicine and dentistry. Hypnosis used for anesthesia was described by the Hindus in their medical writing and much space was given to dental care and treatment with emphasis on brushing and the extraction of bad teeth. The 7th Century B.C. saw the rise and fall of the Assyrian Empire and the destruction of Nineveh, but among the records left is a medical treatise which included fifty-two rules for mouth cleanliness.

In Greece, Hippocrates, an early advocate of prevention, stated that diseases should be combated in their origin. When he talked or wrote about teeth he discussed issues such as irregular formations, the shedding process and the importance of teeth in art forms. He believed that long-lived individuals had a greater number of teeth and that men had more teeth than women. It seems strange that this statement and similar ones of other learned men were accepted for years without question. No one thought to count the number of teeth in a representative number of men and women, a simple, logical procedure which would have disproven the idea.

Several hundred years later Ovid, perhaps more concerned with social niceties than prevention, suggested in his "Art of Love Making" that "the girl who wishes to charm her lover, should not brush her teeth in his presence." Pliny the Elder, a Roman naturalist, discoursed on hygiene of the mouth and the beauty of the teeth, recommending dentifrices to clean and whiten black teeth and suggesting a salt bath as a mouthwash.

The increased leisure time of the upper strata of Roman citizenry encouraged participation in politics, philosophy and natural science. The extra leisure hours also gave the Romans time to be concerned with their personal appearance. History tells us that Roman women cleaned their teeth but, since this was limited to the anterior portions of the mouth, we must conclude that they were more interested in their appearance than personal hygiene and comfort. Patricians of the Empire period of Rome often had special slaves known as *Mastiche*. This name came from the mastic wood sticks they used to cleanse and polish their masters' teeth. Latins called these polishing sticks *Dentiscalpeum* or *Lentiscus* after the name of the wood used.

Marco Polo described the interesting Chinese custom of decorating the teeth with thin plates of gold. These plates, according to his account, were nicely fitted and left on all the time. The covering was placed on the teeth in order to preserve their beauty, although the Chinese believed this was good oral hygiene practice. They cleansed their teeth daily, not to promote health, but because of religious beliefs.

Wars and constant struggle for power and existence did not aid the development of dentistry. By the beginning of the Middle Ages, years 476-1453 A.D., medical and dental knowledge was the property of monks, for only they could read the remaining manuscripts. For some time, assisted by barbers, they had been the surgeons performing most of the extractions of teeth. During the reign of Edward II, the Pope ruled that any operation involving the shedding of blood was not fitting for priests. At that time, barbers, already knowledgeable about certain aspects of the operation, became tooth pullers. The physicians who performed some extractions were greatly relieved and, although they considered barbers as inferiors, were willing to delegate this unpleasant task. By 1308 barbers were incorporated by royal order as a Guild. Competitors were vagabond "tooth drawers" who plied their trade on street corners or at county fairs.

During the Middle Ages the body and its physical care were not very important to the ordinary man, for the Church taught him that sensuous enjoyment was sinful: it was wrong to gaze at another's body, or even his own. There were people, however, who cared about physical comfort. Some men used the point of a knife after eating, while still seated at the table, to remove fragments of food from between their teeth. This custom so offended Cardinal Richelieu that he ordered that the tips of all knives be blunted, and even today the tips of our table knives are rounded. Erasmus, a Dutch scholar of the Middle Ages, was offended by crude people who used a napkin or the tablecloth for wiping their teeth after dining and so recommended rinsing the mouth with water as a substitute, and Giovanni della Casa, an Italian contemporary writer, suggested drinking wine for tooth and mouth cleansing rather than using the tablecloth.

At the beginning of the 15th Century dental health was the subject of many writers. Giovanni of Arcoli gave a detailed list of hygiene rules for preservation of the teeth. He suggested that the patient should avoid indigestion; that excessive movement after eating was harmful, as was vomiting; that sweet or viscous food should not be eaten; that extremes of temperature were harmful to the teeth; that after meals the teeth should be cleansed with slivers of wood (astringent wood such as cypress, aloes, pine, rosemary, juniper) and rubbed with a suitable dentifrice.

Early mouthwashes and dentifrices were not rational combinations of ingredients, but were concocted solely according to superstitious custom or the imagination of the physician or priest. It seemed that the more ingredients used the more efficacious the resultant mixture became. Herbs were important as medicinal or flavoring agents, and were often used empirically, but the use of ground parts of animals and human urine were uneducated attempts to achieve the impossible. The lack of understanding of the actions and reactions of these potions did little harm but did not arrest dental decay, periodontitis or other dental diseases. The usefulness of these preparations was believed to be influenced by the manner of finding and preparing the ingredients. Some items were to be found only by moonlight, others were to be hidden from moonlight. The magnificent claims of today's manufacturers are almost as unbelievable as those of yesteryear, and the wish for "magic potions" has not lessened to any marked degree today.

Toothpicks, chewsticks, and a rag wrapped around the finger are early examples of toothbrushes. At first, any pointed stick sufficed as a toothpick, but as early as 1300 B.C. toothpicks were made in fancy shapes, formed in precious metals and jeweled; some of them doubled as ear picks or fingernail cleaners. Containers for toothpicks were highly prized as ornaments and up to the 17th Century were worn around the neck or on belts. A toothpick seller on the street was an accepted part of city living as late as 1780. Sarsaparilla is still a favored chewstick in parts of the United States and people in many countries use such sticks routinely.

Although the Chinese had toothbrushes by 1498, a prisoner in an English jail is credited with inventing the first toothbrush. We are deeply indebted to him for an efficient way of freeing our teeth of food debris and plaque. Toothbrushes of all sizes and shapes have been preserved throughout the years so that we can trace their family history from the early Chinese brush to those of the present day.

The blind submission to tradition during the Middle Ages came to a halt starting with Martin Luther's defiance of Papal encyclicals. Not only were religion and morals scrutinized but science, too, was questioned. What had once been accepted unequivocally was now reexamined and sometimes found lacking a sound foundation.

The Renaissance brought a revival of writing and textbooks. Much serious writing which was not religious was directed toward the teeth and their care. Early researchers in dental anatomy were Leonardo da Vinci, Andreas Vesalius and Fallopius, all of whom accurately recorded their findings. Leonardo da Vinci made biological studies in masticatory musculature, the nerve supply of the teeth, dental anatomy and occlusion, drawing and describing the teeth and their relationships. Andreas Vesalius' description of general anatomy was excellent and he is generally known as the founder of the science of anatomy. He described the deciduous tooth system and articulation of the teeth. His treatises on the teeth were similar to da Vinci's, but not as accurate. Fallopius did some accurate research on the development of the teeth and discovered that each tooth bud was encased in a separate follicle.

Avicenna wrote much about prophylaxis and the preservation of the teeth, attaching importance to them and warning his readers that abrasive dentifrices damaged the teeth. Abulcasis, the father of periodontia, advised the use of salt water as a mouth rinse and gave tartar serious consideration, recommending removal of these deposits by scraping. He advised fourteen scalers of different shapes for this procedure; by placing the patient's head on his knees, he performed this service for him. If necessary the process was repeated each day until the teeth lost their dirty color.

Until 1530 when the first book devoted entirely to dentistry was published, dentistry had always been included with medicine. Early dentists were called toothers or tooth workers, then Guy de Chauliac used "dentista" in a 1363 manuscript, and Pierre Fauchard in 1728 was the first to use "dentist."

During the early part of the 17th Century, although the church disapproved, Galileo and others were investigating the heavens and the part the earth played in the solar system. By the later part of the century the Dutch naturalist Anton van Leeuwenhoek was using the microscope, opening the way for new discoveries in medicine and dentistry. The ever-changing climate of opinion was soon to allow anatomists and physiologists to perform dissection on the human body and thus to substitute positive knowledge for guesswork.

A definite and continuous history of dentistry begins in the early 18th Century. Dentists of that period were artisans, not scholars, and because they were jealous of their craft they did not keep records. The first practitioner, therefore, is unrecorded, but there is ample proof that Europeans, Arabians and South Americans worked on teeth. In the Old World only prosthesis was attempted, but South American Indians practiced operative dentistry, restoring individual teeth through artificial means.

Early Dentistry in the United States

The Separatists who came to Massachusetts in 1630 brought three barber surgeons with them. One account says the Plymouth Company sent a physician, an apothecary, three barber surgeons and "these were medically educated gentlemen who confined their practice to treating diseased conditions of the teeth and gums, correcting irregularities, cleaning and filling the teeth, extracting and replacing with artificial substitutes."

The advent of the printing press made it possible to circularize some segments of the population and advertise the possibilities of dental care. Pamphlets and books on the subject of dentistry soon followed as a natural outgrowth. Dental advice from the cradle to the grave was provided in 1804 by M. N. DuBois De Chemant "formerly Surgeon of Paris, residing now in London" who published a "Dissertation on Artificial Teeth, Including Advice to Mothers and Nurses on Prevention and Cure of These Diseases Which Attend the First Dentition."

It is uncertain whether John Baker or Robert Woofendale was the first qualified dentist to practice in the United States, but it is known that Baker was a "Friend," probably born in England, who lived in Cork before going to Jamaica and then to Boston. He was one of the early benefactors of education, willing his property to what is now Trinity School. John Baker, M.D., taught Paul Revere, Isaac Greenwood and H. Josiah Flagg the art of dentistry. When Baker left Boston, Paul Revere took over his practice. Isaac Greenwood, an ivory turner as well as a dentist, was a pioneer in America advising toothbrushes and dentifrices to remove tartar in its first state; he assured the public that no dentifrice whatever will remove it when it becomes a petrified scale.

The November 23, 1780 edition of the Newport, Rhode Island *Mercury* carries the advertisement of John Templeman who offers: "Scaling the teeth, is to take from them an infectious tartar, which destroys the enamel, eats the gums, gives the scurvy, and frequently causes the teeth to drop out." The advertisement also illustrates the earliest attempt in this country to regulate children's teeth and to use crowns on teeth. He made an attempt to educate the public to good dental care and did not try to mislead them as many less trained practitioners did.

Growing pains were besetting dentistry on all sides. At that time all dentists were trained in an office by a practitioner because there were no dental schools. The length of time and the quality of instruction were far from being uniform and there were no controls on dental practice except that of public acceptance. There were, of course, charlatans as well as conscientious dentists. The poorly qualified but orthodox dentist could be coped with but some individuals created serious problems for the best practitioners of the time.

Among these unorthodox dentists were two Frenchmen, the Messrs. Crawcour, who came to New York City in 1834 and advertised a radically different, more comfortable way of treating dental caries. The accepted technique of the day was to remove decay by hand, then fill the cavity with gold foil. The Crawcours announced that they could avoid the discomfort of the usual treatment by using "Royal Mineral Succedaneum," an amalgam of silver and mercury, not too scrupulously prepared. Apparently they made no cavity preparation and there were objections from all sides to the use of mercury which was poisonous to the human system. Because the mixture of silver and amalgam was carelessly prepared the filling material expanded, causing discomfort, or shrunk, in which case the filling fell out. Placing any filling over decay is disastrous, so with more than one good reason legitimate dentists of the day opposed these charlatans.

As the clientele of the most respected practitioners left them for these French upstarts the leaders of the dental profession in New York City realized they must take action. The result was that the Society of Surgeon Dentists of the City of New York was organized to "promote the respectability of the profession, by putting down if possible of all imposition and unprincipled quackery, by which the public and the profession at large are made to suffer." An auxiliary association in western New York was formed but, as the problem of the Crawcours disappeared, so did the Society of Surgeon Dentists.

The filling material that these charlatans had introduced still had influence, for even the poorest operator could manipulate it. In 1839 Solymon Brown wrote "I am pained to hear that this execrable material (amalgam) is still used by some unprincipled men in this country." This was not the only type of quackery, for reports were made on "mesmerism, fabulous dentifrices and the treatment of ailing teeth by steam dentistry, using smoke, vapor, or even true steam."

By 1830 there were about three hundred dentists in the United States. More and better instruments were available and it was possible to inform the public regarding care of the teeth. Instead of providing dental care, physicians began to refer patients to those making dentistry a specialty.

Dental Periodicals, Education and Organization

Dentistry then began to grow as a profession. Its dedicated practitioners worked toward the establishment of professional literature to disseminate correct principles and expose error; the establishment of special schools for dental education; and the establishment of professional guilds. These dental pioneers even considered legislation, but the times were not yet ready for this step.

The movement for forming a dental association depended on communication, not only among its members but in apprising the public of new discoveries and proper procedures of professionals. Spooner, in 1838, gave his prescription for elevating the profession: means to inform the community on dental surgery, to convince people of its utility, and to enable them to discriminate between a scientific dentist and a charlatan. He also urged that a semi-annual or quarterly publication be established. Prior to this time all dental articles had been included in medical publications which could no longer afford to give space to dental literature.

The establishment of *The American Journal of Dental Science* probably took place in the home of Solymon Brown in May 1839. Finances were an important factor and the problem was temporarily solved by securing guarantors among the leading dentists, thus enabling publication to continue on a sporadic basis. June 1839 was the date of the specimen number and by 1841, when the first volume neared completion, there were 348 subscribers.

By this time, both medical and dental publications were prophesying that formal training of physicians and dentists would soon be appreciated by the public. Successful dentists had found it lucrative to tutor aspirants to the profession and were not eager to have dental schools established, but respected men such as Horace H. Hayden, who lectured to medical students at the University of Maryland in 1837, and Eleazar Parmly encouraged their establishment. Chapin A. Harris was also active in the movement; he received his license from the Maryland Medical and Chirurgical Faculty in 1833 after having been trained earlier in medicine and dentistry by his brother, John, a physician with special interest in dentistry, in Bainbridge, Ohio. Harris contributed to the literature of his profession and, as editor of *The American Journal of Dental Science,* urged collegiate dental education and promoted formation of a dental organization. Efforts of the leaders of dentistry were rewarded when a charter was granted for establishment of the Baltimore College of Dental Surgery with Harris as dean of this first dental college.

Formal dental education proved successful in a few short years, but practitioners realized that there still must be some distinction between qualified and unqualified dentists and soon proposed licensing procedures. Alabama formulated the first law regulating the practice of dentistry and quickly reported that it had failed to cure the ills it aimed for. The examiners were physicians who often knew nothing about dentistry, and the public was opposed to legislation restricting access to any occupation. Solymon Brown then proposed that, if there were to be no legislation, dentists should form an organization so that the power of numbers could be brought to bear on goals to be accomplished. In the summer of 1840 fifteen prominent dentists met in New York City and formally organized the American Society of Dental Surgeons. The first society was well founded but, due to physical difficulties of transportation and communication and the rivalry between the East and the West, it declined, finally dying in 1850.

Chapin Harris in August of 1841 offered the *American Journal* as the official voice of the American Society of Dental Surgeons. Other periodicals soon appeared, among them the *Dental News Letter* (1847) of the dental supply firm of Jones, White and Company, forerunner of the S. S. White Company, and *Dental Items of Interest*. The *Dental News Letter* merged with *Dental Cosmos,* which was the leading journal here and abroad until 1936 when it merged with the *Journal of the American Dental Association.* Both the *Dental Register of the West,* a publication of the Mississippi Valley Association, and the *American Journal of Dental Science* urged education of the public in preventive measures and by 1841 educational literature was published and distributed.

While politicians argued the pros and cons of slavery and the South threatened secession, dentists were concerned with uniting dentistry by replacing the existing pseudo-national associations with a new national association with a membership representative of organized dentistry. These men sincerely believed that such an organization could further the scientific standing of dentistry, scientific knowledge and techniques, protect and educate the public, and encourage formation of local and regional societies. They were vocal and convincing and, as a result, the American Dental Association as we know it was formed in 1859.

From 1860 to 1912 the American Dental Association endeavored to become representative of American dentistry. In addition to its original objectives it encouraged preliminary dental education, the advancement of dental education and licensure and scientific research. Despite the high goals and the dedication of its members, it was not until 1897 that the Southern Dental Association and the American Dental Association became one under the name of the National Dental Association. Later reorganization took place and the objectives of the Association broadened to include much wider interests of the profession. The spirit of patriotism during World War I fostered the movement to change the Association name back to the American Dental Association.

With freedom granted to the American Negro, even the minimum dental care given him became almost non-existent. A few, who had been laboratory mechanics, learned dentistry through apprenticeship. When dental schools were established in 1840 the Negro was denied entry, but Howard University Dental School included one among its first six graduates in 1867.

By 1890 local groups of colored dentists had formed and the first dental organization of ethical colored dentists, begun as the Washington Society of Colored Dentists, was the R. T. Freeman Dental Society of the District of Columbia, named in honor of the first graduate. As interest grew these societies expanded, progressing from a three-state alliance to an Inter-State Dental Association to a national group formed in 1932. With the release of the name by the American Dental Association it became the National Dental Association of today. Patterned after the structure of the ADA, local and regional groups have formed study clubs, established clinics for the indigent, cooperated with state health boards and evidenced lasting interest in Meharry and Howard Dental Schools.

Because the Association represents the majority of dental practitioners, it has cooperated with associations of dental examiners and dental faculties in setting up relatively uniform requirements for dental education, preliminary educational requirements and the establishment of national board examinations. Another challenge to organized dentistry was scientific research. For years the limited amount of research was performed mainly in dental schools or by various individuals, but in the mid-twenties the Bureau of Standards was able to initiate a cooperative program for Association-sponsored fellowships. A fellowship at the National Institutes of Health eventually led to the founding of the National Institute of Dental Research as one of the National Institutes of Health.

Early Dental Hygiene

In fulfilling its obligation to the public, dentistry has stressed the value of oral health care. This in part has led to the need for more trained dental auxiliaries. Dental hygiene was established in the early years of this century when stress was placed on dental care for school children. The dental hygienist was trained to provide principles of mouth hygiene, nutrition and good health practices as well as to scale and polish the teeth.

The first dental periodical in this country, *The American Journal of Dental Science,* in 1844, five years after its inception, printed an editorial entitled "Dental Hygiene." The unrecorded writer, who was undoubtedly one of the three editors, Chapin Harris, Edward Maynard or Amos Wescott, deplored the fact that so much attention was given to mechanical dentistry and surgery and that the "hygiene of the teeth [was] almost wholly neglected." The editorial continued: "Certainly there is no part of the physical organism of which prevention of disease can be more successfully or effectually applied than to those organs [the teeth]." The approved procedure recommended by Parmly, one of the first to give a paper on educating the public in dental care, followed. The procedure consisted of using waxed floss silk four or five times a day, by which method the patient could keep his teeth clean. He suggested that pamphlets giving correct information and encouraging dental hygiene be distributed through the American Society of Dental Surgeons. This first effort toward oral hygiene placed the responsibility directly on the patient.

"Prophylaxis, or Prevention of Dental Decay," published in 1870, was written by a New Orleans Dental College professor, Andrew McLain, who promoted diet and mouth care. Others in this period referred to the diet as an important factor in relation to diseases of the teeth and gums but no emphasis was given to cleaning the teeth. Mills of Brooklyn wrote an article in 1879 in which he described the need to keep the teeth cleaned and polished but did not offer any specific instructions or procedures. However, his article is noteworthy since it seems to be the first one to mention the dental explorer.

By 1844 Rhein of New York City advocated that dentists should make pupils of their patients and teach them how to brush their teeth effectively; he also proposed that the Board of Education promote a program of oral hygiene for school children. That same year Rhein gave a paper on "Oral Hygiene" in which he commented that the subject of oral hygiene was commonly overlooked because it seemed so simple. However, he said, most patients do not know how to maintain a healthy mouth condition. To him, this condition was of vital importance and he was encouraged by the frequency with which the subject was being considered by dental societies. Rhein believed that all patients, not just a chosen few, should be instructed in mouth care. The principal article necessary for this care, he stated, is the toothbrush, but the public knew neither how to brush properly nor how to choose a good toothbrush. He then gave directions for a thorough brushing technique and recommended using a waxed dental floss to clean between the teeth.

Another pioneer in public health dentistry was Robert Robin Andrews. In 1897 he submitted to the *Journal of the American Medical Association* a strong plea for the enactment of a law that would require the examination of the mouths and teeth of the children in public schools. He recommended that a committee from the dental societies petition the Board of Education to appoint an examining dentist to each school and ask for the complete cooperation and support of every dental organization in the country.

Interest continued to develop in dental hygiene and in the need of the public to have clean mouths, the South being particularly active in the matter of public education. As long ago as 1887 the Alabama Dental Association adopted a resolution acknowledging the responsibility of the dental profession to inform the public of the advantages to be derived from proper dental hygiene and proposed that "a practical lecturer should be employed, and instructed to visit our schools, both public and private, and deliver lectures of a plain and simple character to the pupils, instructing them in the proper care for the teeth."

4

"Prophylaxis in the Field of the Dental Surgeon" was the title of a paper presented by Atkinson of New York City in 1890. Perhaps he was ahead of his time, for he accurately envisioned the scope of dental prophylaxis. To quote him:

Prophylaxis presents four closely related and two attendant aspects of consideration:

1. Prevention, properly a broad effort of education to teach to avoid.
2. Diet, a means of preparation of the system to assist prevention.
3. Hygiene, a regulation of circumstances closely governing [prevention].
4. Regimen, ruling of use of system, food, article and circumstance under the instruction of the preceding aspects; add to these, operative and medicinal interference in the progress of disordered and diseased conditions, and the breadth of prophylaxis is before us.

Many dentists visualized and hoped for preventive dentistry, but it was D. D. Smith of Philadelphia who began a preventive practice in 1894. With forceful, convincing arguments and demonstrations he tried to impress the dental profession with the importance of this treatment. Smith first treated members of his family and a few patients, proving during a four-year period that decay prevention and mouth health were possible through this care. He spoke to many dental groups and exhibited his patients to them in his office. It is the consensus that Smith is truly the father of dental prophylaxis for, while others followed this plan, he was the first to present a definite system of dental prophylaxis, to share his technique with the profession and to show clinical results in his patients' mouths.

Smith was insistent that correct diet provided a foundation for good teeth. He stressed the importance of a clean mouth as the proper environment for clean teeth, "free from the paralyzing effects of external deposits." Believing as he did that it takes more than "brushing, germicidal washes, soaps or dentifrices," he recommended polishing with an orangewood stick and fine pumice. He suggested that mothers be instructed in caring for their children's teeth, polishing the deciduous teeth once a week, and that adults' teeth be polished once in three or four weeks. In his paper he outlined nutritional requirements of people of various ages, and under hygiene and regimen discussed bathing, clothing and home dental care procedures. Smith pointed out that prophylaxis was more than cleaning the teeth. "The filling of teeth and their extraction and treatment, are all prophylactic as defending from more serious consequences. . . ." He believed nurses should be taught to care for their patients' mouths.

In 1901 Smith presented another paper "Oral Prophylaxis," in which he differentiated "cleaning the teeth" from his system of prophylactic treatment. He listed differences in methods, extent and thoroughness of the operation, frequency of treatment and "objectives sought and results obtained—the prevention both of decay and pyorrhea." He recommended the use of scalers and thorough hand polishing of all exposed surfaces for he thought power polishers should never be used. He believed that the polishing action of pumice used with a porte-polisher stimulated the tooth, benefitting it in its entirety as well as improving the gums and alveolar structure.

First Women in the Field of Dentistry

Dentistry, reluctant to accept women in its ranks, greeted the idea with amusement mixed with indignation, but by 1869 two women had been accepted as students in separate dental colleges. It was suggested that women might be assistants to dentists and that when they had worked in the office and learned some procedures they might work on deciduous teeth and take over the "regulating of teeth."

The first suggestion for training women to clean teeth seems to have come from C. M. Wright of Cincinnati, Ohio, who presented "A Plea For A Subspecialty in Dentistry" in 1902. Smith's paper which advocated the careful polishing of teeth throughout life had reenforced Wright's idea and he felt impelled to present suggestions on a subspecialty of dentistry devoted to the polishing of the teeth and the massage of gums. He suggested that these operators be educated women of refinement, that they be trained in dental colleges and that after one year of study and practice and satisfactory evidence of proficiency they be granted a certificate of competence. They could then be "employed by dentists for this special work, or may practice at parlours of their own, or at the homes of patients, the dentists using their influence and recommending the new specialists . . ."

Wright realized that dentistry as a profession had neglected the operations of carefully and routinely scaling and polishing the teeth. He knew the quick operation done with wheels and brushes with the electric engine was only for esthetic effect and that most dentists, realizing the value of proper care, would be glad to have this work done by experts. He stated that about twenty-five years previously (1877) he had suggested this to a young woman and, because he was convinced that it was an excellent idea, again to another young lady who had to abandon the idea because there appeared no way to secure this type of training. He felt that this subspecialty field of dentistry would place dentistry on a higher plane, and in a few years would do more for the human family than toothpaste or powder or other restorative measures.

Naturally, fears were expressed that a partially educated subspecialist would engage in the illegal practice of dentistry. Wright was prepared with arguments and suggested, among other things, that laws controlling the dentist could be modified to allow the practice of these new specialists, laws which would control and limit them. He believed that women would remain within the scope of their training.

Around the turn of the century Thaddeus P. Hyatt, sometimes known as the father of preventive dentistry, tried to convince his fellow practitioners that educating the public in matters of mouth cleanliness was of paramount importance and would result in higher standards of general health. Hyatt was one of the first dentists in New York to encourage acceptance of the dental hygienist for he believed that dentistry should not only repair teeth but should help avoid the need for repair.

That same year F. W. Low of Buffalo, New York, proposed a new profession, that of odontocure; a woman with an orangewood stick and pumice would go to patients' homes to polish their teeth. In 1903 Rhein twice presented a paper on "The Dental Nurse" which gave impetus to the cause of using a dental aide, as a consequence of his prominence in the profession.

As had been done before, he pointed out the need for prophylactic services, outlining why the procedure was neglected as well as its beneficial results. Rhein may have been one of the earliest physicians to point to the permissiveness of the medical profession in allowing the trained nurse to perform so many services and the restrictiveness of the dental profession in not allowing specially trained dental nurses to be employed.

The possibility of using dental graduates for this prophylactic work was discussed, but it was admitted that the graduate with any ambition would not want to remain in this restricted field for any length of time. It was agreed that suitable female assistants would have many advantages to the profession. Rhein, after outlining the extent of their training, advocated licensing examinations by the state board of dental examiners and that these women be allowed to work only under the prescription of the patient's dentist.

The subject had been introduced by Rhein at New Orleans before the Stomatological Section of the American Medical Association which endorsed his plan with the hope that it would lead to amendment of dental laws so that the appointment and employment of dental nurses would be legalized. Rhein concluded his paper with three reasons why his plan should be approved:

First. It will tend materially toward the public good.
Second. It will open to womankind a new vocation second to none in desirability.
Third. It will materially aid the stomatologist in the quality of his results.

The New York State Dental Society was impressed with these proposals and offered a resolution recommending that their Legislative Committee work on amending the existing dental law to conform with the views expressed by Rhein. Through his efforts and the support of prominent dentists, New York, in 1916, legalized the dental nurse.

Dr. Fones and Dental Hygiene

Immediately after graduating from the New York College of Dentistry in 1890, Alfred Civilion Fones returned to his birthplace, Bridgeport, Connecticut, to practice dentistry with his father. After hearing Smith and seeing some of his patients, he became convinced of the value of prevention and decided to incorporate this new concept into his practice. Fones immediately recognized one of the problems as that of office time. On the trip home from Smith's Philadelphia office he suggested to his traveling companion, William Jarvie, that a woman might be trained to do this prophylactic work so that the dentist would be free to continue his operative procedures. During the following years Fones perfected his technique of scaling and polishing and taught his patients how to perform necessary home care procedures. By 1906 the beneficial changes in his practice were evident when compared to his father's practice which had remained unchanged. Because he was so intensely interested in the subject of prevention, Fones accepted a position at the New York College of Dental and Oral Surgery to lecture on dental prophylaxis, and he presented numerous papers and clinics on his technique.

Many dentists incorporated these principles into their dental practices, but in so doing found that preventive services and patient instruction were time consuming and could not be performed in the ideal sense because of the demand for operative work. Beginning in 1899 Fones, who was to become known as the father of dental hygiene, had followed Smith's principles and by 1901 had worked out a system in his own office. He, too, had found it was not feasible to carry out all these necessary procedures himself, so in 1906 he trained his assistant, Irene Newman, to practice this specialty.

Contrary to the accepted facts, Mrs. Newman may not have been the first dental hygienist, although she may well have been the first licensed dental hygienist. The dental assistant of C. M. Wright was trained to perform these procedures at an early but unknown date. Additionally, newly discovered information changes another fact, that Fones established the first courses for dental hygienists. His was the first to continue, but the Ohio College of Dental Surgery should be credited with conducting the first formal training course for dental hygienists and dental assistants. This course, given in 1910-1911, was discontinued after one year because of the strong and bitter opposition of Ohio dentists. Fones' course began in 1913 and its first group of young ladies graduated in 1914.

Connecticut amended its dental law in 1907 to make it unlawful for dentists to employ unlicensed assistants in their offices, and Fones, the chairman of the Connecticut Dental Association Legislative Committee, proposed a modifying clause so that this amendment "shall not prevent an assistant of a registered or licensed dentist from performing the so-called operation of cleaning teeth." This was the first dental law provision ever made to allow performance of prophylactic treatment by an operator specially trained and limited who was not a graduate dentist.

Fones outlined a course of study for Mrs. Newman so that she would have both some basic dental and science background as well as the mechan-

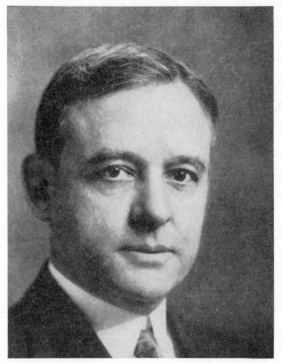

Figure 1. Alfred Civilion Fones, the Father of Dental Hygiene. (Courtesy of the Fones School of Dental Hygiene, Bridgeport, Connecticut.)

ical skills necessary to the scaling and polishing procedures. To begin with, he gave her drawings and books so that she could study the anatomy of the teeth and their surrounding tissues. Natural teeth were secured from a specialist in extracting and were mounted in their normal positions in modeling compound. Next Fones smeared their surfaces with a moist indelible pencil and instructed Mrs. Newman to remove these stains with an orangewood stick and wet pumice. Then one lunch hour she sat in the dental chair and with a mirror watched Fones polish her own teeth. As he worked he explained the finger rests necessary to secure pressure and prevent slipping. Before long, with a mirror in his hand, Fones became the "victim" and Mrs. Newman polished his teeth. At the end of a month of training Fones felt Mrs. Newman was competent to polish the teeth of children. Instruction in the use of instruments followed, using plaster of Paris and varnish on extracted teeth.

Fones continued to present papers emphasizing the dentists' and patients' disregard for oral hygiene and the underlying causes for such disregard. He knew that the dentist must first practice prophylaxis and become an educator in his office before patients can benefit. He believed that 80 per cent of all dental operations could be prevented by teaching and following prophylactic procedures; thus, dental practice would change from one of disease to one of health.

From experience he realized that a busy dentist could not incorporate this preventive service in his practice without aid, so he promulgated the idea of training a woman to be an assistant for this work. He stated "a woman is willing to confine her energy and skill to this one form of treatment. A woman is apt to be conscientious and painstaking in her work. She is honest and reliable, and in this one form of practice, I think, she is better fitted for the position of prophylactic assistant than is a man."

The concept of a female dental assistant was in its pioneer stage and Dr. Fones knew that these assistants would have to be trained in private offices until the demand for their services would induce colleges to establish special courses. He had thought of the possibilities for securing such an assistant: a woman who has been an assistant in the office; a trained medical nurse; the possibility of establishing prophylactic treatments in public schools and the consequent training of young women for this work. Later the profession could be supplied from these clinics. Then he told how he had trained Mrs. Newman and how he would propose to train other types of women. He also had plans for a school clinic staffed by two dentists and thirteen women to give prophylactic treatment and dental health instruction to the children.

H. S. Seip, president of the Pennsylvania State Dental Society, supported the concept of women as prophylactic assistants and mentioned the inability of the dental profession to care for the pressing necessity for treatment of dental caries and irregularities. Thus, he recommended a change in dental laws to license the dental nurse to assist and to be permitted to give prophylactic or surface treatment of teeth. He suggested that training courses should be taught at dental colleges. Rhein agreed with Seip that prophylaxis is not so difficult and that an assistant can learn to perform this service. While Smith agreed with the recommendations of Seip, he disagreed with Rhein for he believed that prophylaxis is one of the most difficult duties of the dentist to perform. Fifty-five years later there is still a controversy, although there is general agreement that the dentist cannot perform all the dentistry that needs to be done and that auxiliary personnel must be delegated more duties and responsibilities.

The elder Fones set an example for his son not only in professional activities but in civic activities as well. Consequently, it is not surprising that when young Fones had proof of the benefits of his own preventive program his thoughts turned to dental health education for children; the public schools were a logical place to begin.

Almost simultaneously Rhein, Fones, Wright, Hyatt and Low, all prominent dentists in different areas of the United States, were talking and writing about women prophylactic workers. Although these four men had not met each other, their concepts were similar, and each man was trying to convince other practitioners of the value of this proposed auxiliary. Fones gives credit to Wright for being "the first one to have properly visualized the dental hygienist as we know her today."* If Fones was not the first to put this idea into action he was the most determined and saw it become a reality.

It was Fones' stated belief that more time and money were being spent on cure than on prevention of dental disease. He observed that the physically poor were unable to cope with any part of daily living and that, since decayed teeth outranked all other physical defects combined in school children, the public schools were the place to start a massive educational program. Many new fillings were needed, but carious lesions, he said, would continue to recur if education was not included in the treatment. It is easy to see that his next step from this line of thought was to undertake to interest the Bridgeport School Board, of which he was a member, in providing such preventive service for their school children rather than the usual relief and repair clinics.

Bridgeport School Dental Health Plan

Through personal experience many of Fones' patients were already indoctrinated with his concepts of oral hygiene and would gladly have furnished the money necessary for him to carry out his prospective school program. He thought it was important that people do something for themselves, so he sought the approval of the Board of Education and an appropriation of funds. Fones wanted the Board of Education to sponsor his program rather than the Board of Health, for he believed education, not restoration, was the real problem.

Several dentists, as a demonstration of the value of dental care, each restored the mouths of ten children and gave them instruction in home care. Teachers of these children reported changes in the boys' behavior and learning after the dental restorations had been placed. Hyatt, Rhein and Palmer, all influential dentists, at Fones' request talked to public gatherings in Bridgeport, urging that the project be implemented.

Through this sincere concern of Fones for the children of Bridgeport, and after four years of intensive work, his plan was approved by the Board of Education to start in 1914. This plan, which he hoped would encompass five years to demonstrate what could be accomplished by using known methods of prevention of dental caries, was the first dental hygiene service in the area of dental public health. The sum of $5,000 was granted and, at his insistence, Fones was put in charge of the program.

* Fones, Mouth Hygiene, Philadelphia, Pa., Lea & Febiger, 1927 3rd Ed., p. 327.

THE SCHEDULE OF
FIFTY-ONE LECTURES
TO BE USED AS A TEXT BOOK FOR

THE EDUCATION OF THE
DENTAL HYGIENISTS

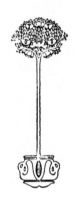

HELD AT 10 WASHINGTON AVENUE
BRIDGEPORT, CONNECTICUT.
COMMENCING NOVEMBER 17th., 1913

A

Schedule of Lectures

Quiz from 7:30 to 8 P.M.
Lectures from 8 to 9 P.M.

NOVEMBER, 1913

Monday,	Nov. 17.	Anatomy—By Raymond C. Osburn, Ph.D.
Thursday,	Nov. 20.	Physiology—By Yandell Henderson, Ph.D. or Alexander Prince, M.D.
Monday,	Nov. 24.	Prof. Osburn.
Friday,	Nov. 28.	Prof. Henderson or Dr. Prince.

DECEMBER, 1913

Monday,	Dec. 1.	Prof. Osburn.
Wednesday,	Dec. 3.	Bacteriology and Sterilization—By L. F. Rettger, Ph.D.
Friday,	Dec. 5.	Prof. Henderson or Dr. Prince.
Monday,	Dec. 8.	Prof. Osburn.
Wednesday,	Dec. 10.	Prof. Rettger.
Friday,	Dec. 12.	Prof. Henderson or Dr. Prince.
Monday,	Dec. 15.	Prof. Osburn.
Wednesday,	Dec. 17.	Prof. Rettger.
Friday,	Dec. 19.	Prof. Henderson or Dr. Prince.
Monday,	Dec. 22.	Prof. Henderson or Dr. Prince.

JANUARY, 1914

Monday,	Jan. 5.	Anatomy and Histology of the Teeth and Jaws—By R. H. W. Strang, M.D., D.D.S.
Wednesday,	Jan. 7.	Prof. Rettger.
Friday,	Jan. 9.	Inflamation—By
Monday,	Jan. 12.	Dr. Strang.
Wednesday,	Jan. 14.	The Skin in Health and Disease—By Dr. G. George MacKee.
Friday,	Jan. 16.	
Monday,	Jan. 19.	Dr. Strang.
Wednesday,	Jan. 21.	Dr. MacKee.
Friday,	Jan. 23.	Oral Secretions—By Edward C. Kirk, Sc.D., D.D.S.
Monday,	Jan. 26.	Dr. Strang.
Wednesday,	Jan. 28.	The Teeth as a Masticating Machine—By Chas. Turner, M.D., D.D.S.
Friday,	Jan. 30.	Dental Caries—By Eugene H. Smith, D.M.D.

FEBRUARY, 1914

Monday,	Feb. 2.	The Chemistry of Food and Nutrition—By Russell H. Chittenden, Ph. D, L.L.D.,Sc.D.
Wednesday,	Feb. 4.	Dr. Turner.
Friday,	Feb. 6.	Dr. Smith.

B

Monday, Feb. 9. Prof. Chittenden.
Wednesday, Feb. 11. Alveolar Abscess By M. L. Rhein, M.D., D.D.S.
Friday, 13 Pyorrhea Alveolaris By R. G. Hutchinson, Jr., D.D.S.
Monday, Feb. 16. Malocclusion By R. Ottolengui, M.D.S.
Wednesday, Feb. 18. Dr. Rhein.
Friday, Feb. 20. Dr. Hutchinson.
Monday, Feb. 23. Dr. Ottolengui
Wednesday, Feb. 25. Dr. Rhein.
Friday, Feb. 27. Deposits and Accretions of the Teeth—By Edward C. Kirk, Sc.D., D.D.S.

MARCH, 1914

Monday, Mar. 2. Dental Prophylaxis—By Alfred C. Fones, D.D.S.
Wednesday, Mar. 4. Factors in Personal Hygiene—By C. Ward Crampton, M.D.
Friday, Mar. 6. The Dental Hygienist as an Assistant in Oral Surgery—By M. I. Schamberg, M.D., D.D.S
Monday, Mar. 9. Dr. Fones.
Wednesday, Mar. 11. Posture and Fresh Air—By Prof. Irving Fisher.
Friday, Mar. 13. The Dental Hygienist as an Assistant in General Practice—By H. E. Chayes, D.D.S.
Monday, Mar. 16. Dr. Fones
Wednesday, Mar. 18. The Teaching of Mouth Hygiene to School Children—By T. P. Hyatt, D.D.S.
Friday, Mar. 20. Dr. Fones.
Monday, Mar. 23. Dr. Fones.
Wednesday, Mar. 25. The Psychology of Handling Children—By Edward C. Kirk, Sc.D., D.D.S.
Friday, Mar. 27. Dr. Fones.
Monday, Mar. 30. Lengthening the Life of the Resistive Forces of the Body—By Dr. William G. Anderson.

This lecture lesson of March 30th will be held in the Yale University Gymnasium, New Haven, Conn.

Commencing Monday, April 6th, there will be a six weeks practical course held five days a week, afternoon and evening sessions. Each student will be required to attend three sessions each week. An effort will be made to arrange with the students for sessions which will prove most convenient for them.

A Baloptican will be used with a reflectiscope, stereopticon and microscope attachment. Pictures may be shown directly from books.

C

Figure 2 A, B, and C. Program of lectures for Dr. Fones' first course in dental hygiene. (Courtesy of The Fones School of Dental Hygiene, Bridgeport, Connecticut.)

The program was divided into four parts:
1. Prophylactic treatment and chart examinations of the mouth.
2. Toothbrush drills and classroom talks on dietetics, mouth hygiene and later general hygiene.
3. Stereopticon lectures for pupils in the higher grades not included in the program.
4. Educational work in the homes by means of special literature for parents and older children.

Grades one through five were included and findings were compared with those of a fifth grade control class which had no mouth hygiene. The incidence of dental caries in the permanent teeth was reduced by 33.9 per cent during the five-year period. Principally this was the result of education and home care. There were no funded repair clinics and only small cavities in first permanent molars of first grade students could be restored by the three school dentists.

The need for trained personnel to carry out the school program became the inspiration for the first course in dental hygiene. To those who knew him Fones was a man of exceptional vision, dedication, perseverance and personality; therefore, he was the ideal person to plan and carry out this inaugural program.

First Course in Dental Hygiene

Considering the special type of service these women were to render, Fones felt that dental nurse was a misnomer for their position. He did not want the name to be associated with disease, but he did want it to be a proper description. A hygienist is one who is versed in the science of health and the prevention of disease, and eventually "dental hygienist" was coined and is still accepted.

Dentists, physicians and educators agreed to share in the teaching responsibilities of this first group of ladies. These instructors came from Universities of Harvard, Yale, Pennsylvania and Columbia College of Physicians and Surgeons, and included prominent specialists from practices in New York and Bridgeport. It was an outstanding faculty but, most remarkable, men of medicine as well as dentistry were giving their time gratis to help create Fones' dream. Through sheer perseverance and sincere belief in his proposal he was able to convince them of the validity of his beliefs in oral hygiene and its many benefits. Their traveling expenses were paid out of his own pocket, but imagine how dedicated they were to spend so many hours travelling to Bridgeport from Philadelphia or Boston. The lectures given by these gentlemen were compiled and became the first dental hygiene textbook, *Mouth Hygiene,* edited by Fones with R. H. W. Strang and E. C. Kirk as associate editors.

With the course of instruction planned and instructors secured, there still remained a classroom and equipment to be found. Fones, his father, and Mrs. Newman occupied offices on the second floor of what had once been the carriage house of his home. The first floor was devoted to a reception room, a secretary's office, rest rooms and a large area sometimes used as a garage. It was this large room which was converted into a classroom, complete with desks, projector and screen for lectures. A part of the costs were underwritten by Fones' wealthier patients who were anxious to support the school.

When the first portion of the course had been covered, the classroom changed its form and became a clinic for practical instruction in prophylactic procedures. This part of the course was given five afternoons and evenings a week and students were required to attend at least three of these sessions. The desks were replaced with fifteen chairs with work tables and cuspidors loaned by the S. S. White Dental Manufacturing Company. A drop light hung over each chair for illumination. In the center of the room was a sink with running hot and cold water and a zinc table large enough for a sterilizer which was a tub of water with a burner underneath. Individual milkshake mixers held instruments to be placed in the tub. Other trays held supplies of pumice for polishing, alcohol for sterilizing mirrors and handles of instruments which could not be placed in boiling water, and other necessary items. Each girl had her own instruments and other equipment, furnished at cost, and a japanned box in which these could be locked.

Mannikins with rubber cheeks, a tongue, movable jaws and a full complement of teeth were attached to the chairs in place of headrests. Students were first taught a system of going over the teeth with instruments and then

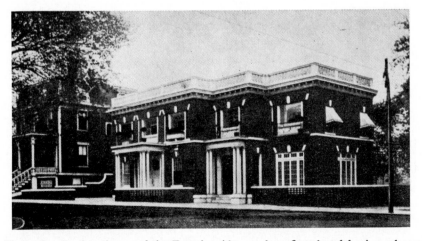

Figure 3. Carriage house of the Fones' residence where first dental hygiene classes were held. (Courtesy of The Fones School of Dental Hygiene, Bridgeport, Connecticut.)

a porte-polisher, then the correct positions for holding instruments, the best fulcrum points and the sequence of the teeth to be cleaned. Just as Mrs. Newman had been instructed, the teeth were thoroughly stained before polishing and artificial calculus was applied for practice in instrumentation. Each student had to pass a rigorous examination at every stage of the work. When the students were proficient enough to treat patients they first worked on children, progressing to treating adults.

Only prophylactic treatment was taught, but this most thoroughly. All surfaces of the teeth were cleaned with the porte-polisher, the interproximal surfaces with dental floss, the occlusals with a brush. Reports on each child patient were made and sent to the school principal. Each child was taught how to brush his teeth and then he demonstrated what he had learned. If he did not bring his own toothbrush, Fones supplied one.

Fones anticipated no problem in recruiting enough young women to enroll in this first course in dental hygiene, since his campaign for a demonstration program in Bridgeport public schools had been well publicized in the newspapers. However, until the money was appropriated no assurance could be given that positions would be available at the end of the course of instruction. Not able to find students, he turned to his profession, and recruited twenty-four assistants from offices of his fellow practitioners, three wives of these dentists, three college graduates who were teaching school and three trained nurses. Tuition was a nominal twenty dollars. Of the thirty-three original enrollees, twenty-seven graduated and were given diplomas on June 5, 1914. Among them were Mrs. Newman and Mrs. Fones.

Because of the uncertainty of activation of the public school program many of the girls had accepted positions in private offices. Two of the class, however, were employed as supervisors and they assisted in recruiting and training other students for school work. Ten young ladies about to graduate from Bridgeport High School were interested in taking an intensive summer course in theory and practice. It was merely an introduction for they had to take additional training in order to be eligible for licensure. At least one of these seniors took dental hygiene courses at the same time she finished her high school work.

The dental hygienists in the public schools were paid $1.50 per day, $9.00 a week. Because of the need for dental hygienists two more classes were conducted by Fones before organized institutions took over their education. Among the ninety-seven graduates of Fones' three classes were many who traveled to distant parts of the United States and to Hawaii, pioneering in many areas of dental hygiene. Mrs. Fones often substituted for the hygienists in schools for, as she said, that was one way to get to see her husband.

The first class of dental hygienists had all the qualities associated with any pioneer group: courage, conviction, dedication, enthusiasm, stamina. Many of them worked part of the day before attending classes. At least two

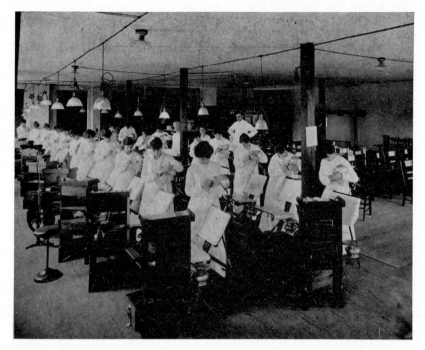

Figure 4. First class of dental hygienists using mannikins for learning scaling procedures. (Courtesy of The Fones School of Dental Hygiene, Bridgeport Connecticut.)

of the girls commuted from fifty-five miles away, a 1½-hour trip by "fast" train, made before and after each class session.

Mrs. Newman was interviewed in 1955 by Frances Dolan, Executive Director of the Fones School of Dental Hygiene, Bridgeport, Connecticut, and Mabel McCarthy, a graduate of one of the original Fones' courses and currently an instructor at Fones School of Dental Hygiene. Mrs. Newman, a second cousin of Fones, became his dental assistant in 1903 and worked with him for nearly thirty years. She said his office was beautiful and there were often visitors who had heard of it and wanted to see for themselves. Some came from as far away as Japan, and the numbers increased after the school was started.

Fones believed strongly in his convictions and concepts and was positive, persuasive, and convincing whether he was talking or writing. It never occurred to him that he was unique; he merely saw the work that needed to be done and did it.

Mrs. Newman, by her account, often gave clinics for Fones, sometimes without warning, as proof of the quality of his training and the effectiveness of the treatment procedures. Once Fones took Mrs. Newman to present a clinic in Massachusetts to furnish positive evidence for the dentists who

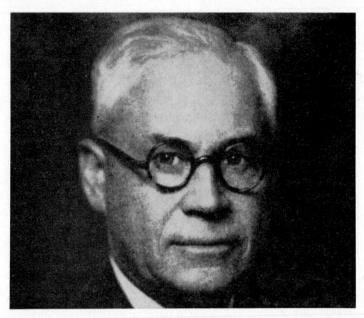

Figure 5. R. H. W. Strang, M.D., D.D.S., Instructor in Anatomy and Histology of the Teeth and Jaws in first course in dental hygiene, and currently Director and Instructor, Fones School of Dental Hygiene, University of Bridgeport, Bridgeport, Connecticut. (Courtesy Fones School of Dental Hygiene.)

were working for dental hygiene licensure in that state. Although opponents pointed to blood on the towel used by the patient as evidence of surgical procedures, the law was enacted, undoubtedly aided by this demonstration.

Fittingly, Mrs. Newman was issued License #1 and became the first president of the first dental hygiene association, the Connecticut Dental Hygienists' Association, which was organized immediately after the graduation of the first class. One of the scholarships awarded by the American Dental Hygienists' Association bears her name.

In September 1915 B. Elizabeth Beatty was hired by the Bridgeport schools and was supplied with portable dental equipment so she could travel from school to school, filling the first permanent molars of the first grade children. Proof of the needs of these children was so great that two more dentists were added to the staff in succeeding years. When funds were needed to continue the dental educational work in the schools there was no problem in securing an appropriation, this time for $10,000, for the 1915-1916 year.

It was necessary to find patients of various types for the dental hygiene students. The results of their work had been so impressive that Boy Scout troops came in groups and some local manufacturers released their employees half an hour early so that they might go to the classroom and have their teeth cleaned.

With the start of World War I, Fones, still concerned with dental needs of the public and realizing the poor condition of most recruits' mouths and the lack of care they certainly would receive when they were sent overseas, did his best to arrange for some kind of dental care for them. Fifty-five dentists of Bridgeport filled as many teeth as possible, and under the leadership of Mrs. Newman in 1917 each member of the Connecticut Dental Hygienists' Association volunteered to clean the teeth of twenty-five soldiers from the nearby army camp. Fones reopened the big classroom and equipped it with twenty dental chairs for their use.

The scope of dental hygiene practice quickly extended beyond private practice and school and in 1915 the state of Connecticut, realizing the possibilities of the profession's future growth, enacted another amendment to the dental law to regulate the practice of these auxiliary workers. For the first time the field of operation of the dental hygienist was legally defined. In so doing, the law set a precedent for the majority of states which later adopted similar laws. This first legal definition of the practice of dental hygiene is as follows:

> Any registered or licensed dentist may employ women assistants, who shall be known as dental hygienists. Such dental hygienists may remove lime deposits, accretions and stains from the exposed surfaces of the teeth and directly beneath the free margins of the gums, but shall not perform any other operation on the teeth or mouth, or on any diseased tissues of the mouth. They may operate in the office of any registered or licensed dentist, or in any public or private institution under the general supervision of a registered or licensed dentist. The dental commission (state board of dental examiners) may revoke the license of any registered or licensed dentist who shall permit any dental hygienist, operating under his supervision, to perform any operation other than that permitted under the provisions of this section.

Massachusetts' dentists tried to introduce a similar amendment into their legislature in 1910 but were unsuccessful until 1915, and New York, as previously mentioned, was not able to enact such legislation until 1916. As soon as the dental hygienist was legalized in these states, three training schools were organized. Louise C. Ball secured a grant of $2,500 from the Rockefeller Foundation and conducted a summer course through Hunter College in 1916. This school became a part of the Vanderbilt Clinic of Columbia University that fall and is a part of the School of Dental and Oral Surgery, Columbia University. The course was a full year in length and required one year of high school for admission to class. A similar school was founded at the Rochester Dental Dispensary, Rochester, New York, under the direction of Harvey J. Burkhart, and another at Forsyth Dental Infirmary for Children, Boston, Massachusetts, with Harold DeWitt Cross as director.

Because dental hygienists fulfilled a very real need, their numbers grew and the graduates spread across the United States. Fourteen schools of dental hygiene were initiated during the thirty years after the first Fones graduating class, with programs designed to meet the needs of local dental practitioners and state licensing boards. As a result of differences in local needs, a variety of courses developed with emphasis on clinical or educational preventive services.

World War II retarded growth of all professional schools. As an aftermath of the war, social consciousness underwent changes and legislators and union leaders proposed or demanded more health care for their constituents. As a result, the need for more dental auxiliary personnel grew. In an attempt to alleviate the shortage of dental hygienists, new programs have been developed throughout the United States. In 1974 there were more than 160 curricula in dental hygiene in operation and more are in planning stages. Currently, more students apply for admission than can be accepted.

All progress depends upon new ideas and the creative application of old ideas, upon the acquisition of further skills and the ability to apply those skills. Dental hygienists must recognize that they stand on the frontier of an era which holds the possibilities of a new Golden Age, in which the general and dental health of the public will be improved and in which, through the extension of educational opportunities, it will be within the power of the individual to develop potential capacities to the maximum. The dental hygienist must recognize also that dentistry today demands continuous learning or the threat of professional deterioration must be faced.

Chronology of Oral Hygiene

B.C.

250,000,000	Animal remains show evidence of traumatic injury of dental origin
100,000,000	Evidence of disease caused by bacterial invasion
100,000	Man contended with retained deciduous teeth, impacted teeth, fractures and rickets
8,000–10,000	Neolithic man practiced knocking out of teeth
5,000	Surgery on the skull performed by Neolithic man Ea, ancient enemy of tooth worm, first deity known to be associated with healing arts
3,500	Toilet set of toothpick, ear scoop and tweezers found in Ningal Temple at Ur
3,000–525	Dentists were specialists of medicine in Egypt Hesi-Ré, Egyptian, earliest known dentist
2,750	Babylonians regulated practice of medicine and dentistry
2,300	Code of Hammurabi written (Babylonia) Toothpicks in use Hindus used hypnosis for obtaining anesthesia
700	Fall of Nineveh, records left included 52 rules for mouth cleanliness
669–626	Ashurbanipal collected first systematic library
469–377	Hippocrates believed disease should be combated in its origin

A.D.

23–79	Pliny the Elder advocated hygiene of the teeth
37–68	Romans had slaves who cleansed their master's teeth
980–1037	Avicenna wrote about prophylaxis and preservation of the teeth
1000	Abulcasis was first writer to give tartar serious consideration
1100	Barbers took over tooth pulling
1254–1372	Marco Polo wrote of gold crowns fabricated by the Chinese
1300–1368	Guy de Chauliac first used "dentista" in a manuscript
1400	Giovanni Arcoli listed rules of hygiene for preservation of teeth Fallopius accurately researched development of teeth
1452–1519	Leonardo Da Vinci studied and described masticatory musculature, nerve supply of the teeth, dental anatomy and occlusion
1498	Chinese made first toothbrush
1514–1564	Vesalius founded the science of anatomy
1530	First book entirely on dentistry, *Artzney Buchlein,* written in German on dental therapeutics
1585–1642	Cardinal Richelieu ordered tips of knives blunted to prevent using them at the table to remove fragments of food from between the teeth
1630	Three barber surgeons came to Massachusetts with Plymouth Company
1632–1723	Anton van Leeuwenhoek by use of microscope discovered microorganisms on teeth
1728	Pierre Fauchard first used "dentist" in a manuscript
1766	John Baker or Robert Woofendale first qualified dentist in United States
1776	Paul Revere made first identification of body based on teeth
1821	Horace Hayden probably lectured medical students on dentistry
1834	Messrs. Crawcour promoted silver and mercury amalgam as filling material Opposition to them encouraged the birth of organized dentistry to protect the public
1839	*American Journal of Dental Science,* first dental periodical in America
1840	Baltimore College of Dental Surgery, first formal dental school Alabama enacted first law regulating practice of dentistry American Society of Dental Surgeons organized
1844	Development of Dental Hygiene begins with publication of editorial, "Dental Hygiene" in *American Journal of Dental Science*
1865	French still believed shape and arrangement of teeth were valid means of judging character
1869	Two women accepted as dental students, Ohio Dental College and Pennsylvania College of Dental Surgery
1870	"Prophylaxis, or Prevention of Dental Decay" published by Dr. Andrew McLain of New Orleans
1879	Dr. G. A. Mills, Brooklyn, stressed need to keep teeth clean and mentioned the use of a dental explorer for the first time

1884   Dr. Meyer L. Rhein (M.D., D.D.S.) of New York City advocated teaching patients to brush effectively and described a model toothbrush

1887   Alabama Dental Association urged that school children be taught to care for their teeth

1890   Dr. C. B. Atkinson described practical benefits of dental prophylaxis

1894   Dr. D. D. Smith began his preventive dental practice

1896   Roentgen ray used in dentistry

1900   Dr. Thaddeus P. Hyatt encouraged acceptance of the dental hygienist

1902   Dr. C. M. Wright, Ohio, first suggested in writing that women be trained to clean teeth, as a subspecialty in dentistry

1906   Dr. Alfred C. Fones, later to be known as the father of dental hygiene, trained his assistant, Mrs. Irene Newman, to be the first dental hygienist

1907   Connecticut amended its dental law to provide for the performance of prophylactic treatment by specially trained operators

1913   First class of dental hygiene students assembled in November
        Name of "dental hygienist" selected by Dr. Fones

1914   First class of dental hygienists graduated in Bridgeport, Connecticut
        First dental hygiene association organized, Connecticut
        Bridgeport, Connecticut instituted first preventive dental hygiene service in public schools

1915   Connecticut first state to define legally the field of operation of the dental hygienist
        Massachusetts amended its dental practice act to allow dental hygienists to practice

1916   New York legalized the dental hygienist
        First textbook for dental hygienists compiled by Dr. Fones
        Three training schools for dental hygienists organized: Hunter College, now Columbia, Rochester Dental Dispensary and Forsyth

1917   First dental hygiene licensure law adopted by Connecticut

References

Atkinson, C. B.: Prophylaxis in the field of the dental surgeon. Int. Dent. J., pp. 371-375, 1891.

Bovic, E. G.: A brief history of the hygiene movement. Chicago Dental Society, February 1942.

Bremner, M. D. K.: *The Story of Dentistry,* 3rd ed. Brooklyn, Dental Items of Interest, 1939.

Bunting, R.: *Oral Hygiene.* Philadelphia, Lea & Febiger, 1954.

Chase, H. S.: Dental hygiene. Trans. Amer. Dent. Assoc., p. 51, 1865.

Dittmar, G. W.: Dental hygienist question in Illinois. Oral Hygiene, 17:1534-1541, 1927.

Dummett, C. O.: *The Growth and Development of the Negro in Dentistry in the United States.* Chicago, National Dental Association, 1952.

Editorial: Dental hygiene. Amer. J. Dent. Sci., 5:244, 1844.

Fones, A. C.: The necessity for and training of a prophylactic assistant. Dent. Cosmos, 54:284-289, 1912.

Fones, A. C.: Origin and history of the dental hygiene movement. J. Amer. Dent. Assoc., 13:1809-1821, 1926.

Fones, A. C.: *Mouth Hygiene,* 3rd ed. Philadelphia, Lea & Febiger, 1927.

Guerini, V.: *History of Dentistry.* Philadelphia, Lea & Febiger, 1909.

Kaufman, J. H.: The dental hygienist and the law. Dent. Outlook, 22:441, 419-422, 1935.

Kingsley, N. W.: Woman—Her position in dentistry. Herald Dent. 3:1, 1884.

Lufkin, A. W.: *A History of Dentistry*. Philadelphia, Lea & Febiger, 1938.

McLain, A.: Prophylaxis or prevention of dental decay. Dent. Reg., 24:158, 1870.

McCarthy, M.: Personal conversation, October 1969.

McCluggage, R. W.: *A History of the American Dental Association*. Chicago, American Dental Association, 1959.

McGehee, W. and Walker, A: *Dental Practice Management,* Chicago, Ill., Year Book Publishers, 1944, p. 123.

Mills, G. A.: How to keep the teeth clean and healthful. Dent. Cosmos, 22:21, 1880.

Newman, I.: Taped interview, August 1955.

Prinz, H.: *Dental Chronology*. Philadelphia, Lea & Febiger, 1945.

Remington, F. L.: Toothbrushes and such. TIC, June 1964, pp. 13-14.

Rhein, M. L.: Oral hygiene. New Engl. J. Dent., 3:356-361, 1884.

Rhein, M. L.: The trained dental nurse. Dent. Cosmos, 45:628-631, 1903.

Smith, D. D.: Prophylaxis in dentistry. Int. Dent. J., 20:22-23, 1899.

Smith, D. D.: Oral prophylaxis. Int. Dent. J., 22:817, 1901.

Smith, M.: *A Short History of Dentistry*. New York, Roy Publishers, 1958.

Strang, R. H. W.: Personal conversation, October 1969.

Weinberger, B. W.: *An Introduction to the History of Dentistry,* Vols. I and II. St. Louis, C. V. Mosby, 1948.

Wright, C. M.: A plea for a subspecialty in dentistry. Int. Dent. J. 23:235, 1902.

Chapter 6

The American Dental Hygienists' Association

The French statesman Tocqueville, who visited the United States in 1840, observed: "Americans of all ages, all conditions, and dispositions constantly form associations. . . . From that moment on they are no longer isolated men but a power from afar whose actions are an example and whose language is listened to." Associations are a vital force in American life, and the American Dental Hygienists' Association is no exception.

An organized group of individuals with similar educational background and interests will stimulate continuing education of its members and improvement of their skills. The group, through its organized efforts, can influence legislation affecting its membership professionally and can help direct the trend of the services they offer. As the demand for health care increases, the activities of the American Dental Hygienists' Association in behalf of its members also increase and become more comprehensive. The Association also offers its members an opportunity to discuss mutual concerns and to exchange information pertinent to the practice of dental hygiene.

First Dental Hygiene Associations

The dental hygienists of Bridgeport, Connecticut, though few in number, formally organized the first association of dental hygienists. The twenty-seven original graduates were going to various parts of Connecticut and wanted to keep in touch with each other as they pioneered this new field. Dr. Fones' enthusiasm lent encouragement for forming an organization, and nineteen charter members and nine associate members accepted the challenge. "The object of this Association shall be to educate the public in, and to advance the cause of Mouth Hygiene for the mutual improvement of its members, and to assist as far as lies within its power in the prevention of disease."* Certainly these young ladies must have dreamed of the day when there would be dental hygienists in every state of the Union and a national association would be established.

Mrs. Irene Newman was elected the first president, and committees were formed to accomplish the work of the organization. Many of the students' non-working hours had been spent with Dr. Fones, bringing a concept of optimum dental health to allied health groups, especially dental societies. The good will and friendliness of the Connecticut Dental Association became evident when they invited the dental hygienists to hold their first state meeting in conjunction with the dentists at Hartford, in April, 1915. In February of that year Mrs. Winifred Hart, secretary, wrote to all members of the Connecticut Dental Association and their wives, inviting them to become associate members, and many accepted the invitation.

At the first state meeting three papers were read by dental hygienists, and ten dental hygienists gave prophylactic treatment and instruction in home care to ten dentists. The interest was so great that the dental hygienists hardly had room to demonstrate. Visiting dentists from New Hampshire and Vermont were so impressed that they invited dental hygienists to bring similar demonstrations the next month to their annual meetings.

Ninety-five members were on the roll by the second annual meeting in New London, Connecticut, where it was announced that dental hygiene had been legalized in New York and in Massachusetts. As the numbers of dental hygienists increased, the need for more definitive legal restrictions became apparent and a legislative committee was appointed to discuss this with the Connecticut State Dental Association.

The fourth annual meeting in New Haven marked the first interchange of ideas among state dental hygiene associations, and schools at Forsyth, Columbia and Rochester sent clinicians. Radiographic techniques were first demonstrated at this meeting, and a report was given concerning the dental care program initiated by Fones and Mrs. Newman for draftees of World War I. The rapid growth of the dental hygiene movement is largely attributable to the complete cooperation of Connecticut dentists.

Formation of a National Organization

As Massachusetts and New York graduated dental hygiene students, they, too, formed state associations. Records show that as more states graduated or licensed dental hygienists, the eastern groups began to consider forming a national association. The idea was dropped because of local

* History of the Connecticut Dental Hygienists' Association. JADHA, 5:26, 1931.

concerns of the moment and the difficulties of communication and transportation.*

Four enthusiastic dental hygienists in California formed a state association in 1919, and by 1920 there were ten active members: two Forsyth graduates, two 1919 graduates and six 1920 graduates of the University of California. Perhaps the great distance and the lack of direct contact with eastern associations stimulated California dental hygienists to consider the need for a national association. In order to promote the ideals of the profession, preserve the rights and interests of its members, and gain strength through mutual cooperation, this small determined group began interesting other states in the formation of a national organization. They suggested that one member from each state dental hygiene association be selected to form a committee to study organization, direct nominations of officers, and draft a constitution and bylaws. Each state group was asked to submit suggestions for a mechanism of organizing this new group.

Guy S. Milberry, Dean of the University of California School of Dentistry and working with California dental hygienists, wrote to Fones. In reply, Fones stated he thought it best for the women to perfect small state and district organizations first. The secretary of an eastern association wrote that they were "babes in the woods and had no business forming a National Association." Such comments did not discourage California dental hygienists; rather, they became more determined.†

Organizational Meeting

During the ensuing year, under the direction of President Elma Platt, California hygienists drafted the following resolution presented by President Platt and Dean Milberry to the House of Delegates of the National Dental Association in June, 1922:

WHEREAS: the Dental Hygienists' Association of California, an organization of graduate licensed dental hygienists with definite purposes in the interest of child health and welfare in particular, and humanity in general, which purposes are similar to those of the dental profession and other health organizations, and
WHEREAS: we, an organized body, are dealing with a common problem, the solution of which depends upon the close cooperation of the dental hygienists with the dental profession, and
WHEREAS: many do not know the professional status of the dental hygienist even though the National Dental Association has officially endorsed the movement;
THEREFORE BE IT RESOLVED: that since our training and practice is common with the practice of dentistry, especially in the educational aspects of preventive dentistry, we respectfully request that the National Dental Association take steps to promote the organization of an American Dental Hygienists' Association,

* History and progress of dental hygiene in the United States. JADHA. 1:3-9, 1927.
† Junck, A., and Barney, E.: A glance backward. No. Calif. State Dent. Hyg. Assoc., 1964.

after the plan of organization of the National Dental Association, which shall become closely associated or affiliated with it for the good of humanity.*

It had been anticipated that this resolution would not be adopted until the following year but, because of enthusiastic support from dentists, it was accepted immediately.

The National Dental Association, which changed its name to the American Dental Association at this meeting, granted dental hygienists conference privileges. The House of Delegates believed it would take too much time for the Dental Association to promote the organization of an American Dental Hygienists' Association and that it was better for dental hygienists to organize themselves as soon as possible. Anita Junck, the new California president, and Elma Platt, Organization Committee chairman, worked with members to plan an organizational meeting in 1923. A constitution patterned after that of the Dental Association was drafted and, after receiving approval from the Dental Association, dental hygienists sent it to other state associations requesting suggestions and corrections.

At the same time, a Conference Committee was appointed with Doctors Anna Hughes, chairman, Harris Wilson, vice-chairman, and members De Witt Cross, Guy Milberry and Alfred Fones; the president and secretary of the ADA, J. P. Buckley and Otto U. King, were included as ex-officio members.

State dental hygiene organizations were invited to send delegates to the national association organizing meeting in September, 1923. New York, Massachusetts, Hawaii and Colorado signified that they favored the constitution drafted by California, and other states indicated they would send delegates.

First Annual Session

The American Dental Hygienist's Association became a reality on September 12, 1923 in Cleveland, Ohio. Forty-six dental hygienists representing the eleven states of California, Colorado, Connecticut, Illinois, Iowa, Massachusetts, Michigan, New York, Ohio, Pennsylvania and West Virginia heard the meeting called to order by W. R. Wright, chairman of the ADA Commission on Mouth Hygiene and Public Instruction.

Dean Milberry read the resolution which the California dental hygienists had presented to the ADA the previous year. Next he quoted from Minutes of the House of Delegates of the ADA indicating their desire to cooperate with the proposed new association:

VOTED, that the recommendation of the Board of Trustees be adopted, That dental hygienists, dental mechanics, and dental assistants, except associations for profit, be encouraged to establish associations in their respective states, and
That they be given conference relations with the ADA, state societies, and subsidiary organizations, the details of which are to be formulated by the Committee on Dental Education in conference.

* Ibid.

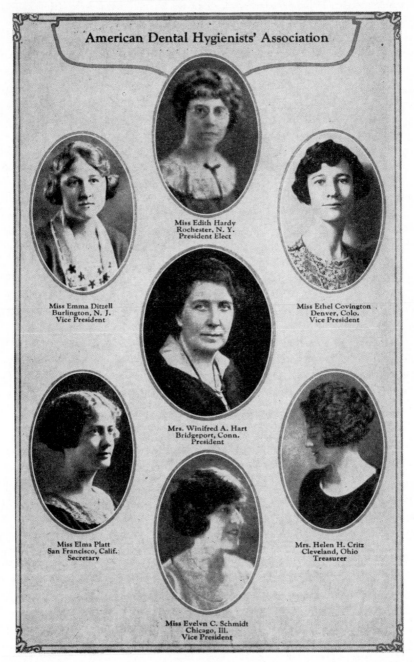

American Dental Hygienists' Association

Miss Edith Hardy
Rochester, N. Y.
President Elect

Miss Emma Ditzell
Burlington, N. J.
Vice President

Miss Ethel Covington
Denver, Colo.
Vice President

Mrs. Winifred A. Hart
Bridgeport, Conn.
President

Miss Elma Platt
San Francisco, Calif.
Secretary

Mrs. Helen H. Critz
Cleveland, Ohio
Treasurer

Miss Evelyn C. Schmidt
Chicago, Ill.
Vice President

Figure 6. First officers of the American Dental Hygienists' Association. (Courtesy A.D.H.A.)

Winifred Hart of Connecticut was voted temporary chairman and Elma Platt of California was voted temporary secretary. Since Miss Platt was not in attendance, Dean Milberry, who had been delegated to represent California dental hygienists, was asked to serve as temporary secretary. On behalf of the ADA Council on Mouth Hygiene and Public Instruction Anna Mims Wright, Mississippi, wife of the Council's chairman, W. R. Wright, presented the new organization with a gavel and their good wishes (Appendix, p. 168).

Though the members in attendance were authorized to represent their state associations, few had official credentials; it was therefore decided that the meeting become open for the consideration of all business. Since the majority of those present had not reviewed the Constitution and Bylaws, portions of them were read. It was agreed that a committee should review these documents during the coming year, giving special attention to financial matters. A committee chaired by Charlotte S. Greenhood, California, was appointed and instructed to send copies to all state associations with the request that they submit any recommendations to the Committee. The Constitution and Bylaws were then adopted provisionally so officers could be elected. Mrs. Winifred Hart, Connecticut, was unanimously elected president, and Edith C. Hardy, New York, president-elect. Evelyn Schmidt, Massachusetts, Emma Ditzell, Pennsylvania, and Ethel Covington, Colorado, became vice-presidents, Elma W. Platt, general secretary, and Helen Hilbish, Ohio, treasurer, to serve with President Hart. Since banks in Cleveland charged $1.00 per month for accounts of less than $100.00 and the new association did not have that much, the treasurer was instructed to carry Association funds in her personal account until further notice.

Growth in Scope and Activities

The first officers of the American Dental Hygienists' Association accepted their responsibilities with excitement and high hopes as well as concern. General members must have been stimulated by the thought of being a part of a new, nationwide professional organization. Some Association officers and committee chairmen are mentioned by name; the limitations of space require that others remain nameless. A book devoted entirely to the history of the American Dental Hygienists' Association could not include all who have contributed significantly to the profession and the Association.

The first meeting was organizational. The second annual meeting of the newly formed Association was held two years later in September, 1925, in Louisville, Kentucky. With the exception of the war years of 1942 and 1945 when travel was restricted, general meetings have been held annually. The business of the second meeting included adoption of a Constitution and Bylaws, election of honorary members and new officers, and reports of constituent activities of the past year given by delegates. Scientific papers by dental hygienists and Dean Milberry were featured. Dental hygienists were invited to attend section meetings of the American Dental Association and an exhibit about dental hygiene was displayed at the dental meeting. Records show that Evelyn Schmidt, a dental hygienist, was employed by the ADA.

Scientific Sessions

At subsequent annual meetings Paul Stillman presented his brushing technique as the program feature one year, William Charters and A. C. Fones described their techniques another year, and three dentists presented a panel-discussion-demonstration at a later session. During the years many distinguished dentists, dental hygienists and members of related professional groups have presented national programs.

George Wandel, Supervisor of the ADA Bureau of Dental Health Education, represented the American Dental Association in welcoming ADHA members to one of its early annual sessions. He suggested standardized school curricula, reciprocity between states, and the establishment of an employment bureau of registration. Whether or not his address was a stimulus, all his recommendations received attention, with varying degrees of success.

W. R. Wright, who called the first meeting to order, sent his compliments to the Association saying that it had grown "to full stature" . . . and admonished the group "to observe the high ethical standards you have maintained. I believe that practically every dentist member of the dental profession considers you indispensable in all mouth health programs" and urged that only those who have the same training be accepted as members.*

The 1926 meeting of the International Dental Congress in Philadelphia was an important occasion. President Edith Hardy presented a paper on dental hygiene read during the IDC meeting. "Ask Me" buttons were worn by dental hygienists who wanted opportunities to talk about their Association while attending the Philadelphia meeting. Six trustees, to be a part of the governing Board of the ADHA, were elected from the general membership.

Exhibits, Table Clinics

In its second year of organization, a poster exhibit and a "health-land" display were prepared by ADHA for display with the Dental Association exhibits. In 1935 a large scrapbook of photographs showing the activities of dental hygienists in private practice, public health, industry, hospitals and training schools was utilized. Some years individual states had dental health exhibits while other years it was a group effort. One exhibit featured dolls dressed in the individual school uniforms, holding ribbons which led to their school on a United States map. The 1940 exhibit was a montage

* Minutes of the ADHA, 1923-1971.

of indoor-outdoor activities of dental hygienists of the United States. The defense program was the incentive for another exhibit which stressed dental health from ages three to twenty-five in "Oral Hygiene Prepares American Youth." In the 1950's the location of schools and the ratio of dentists to dental hygienists were depicted. These first exhibits were designed and constructed by members; in more recent years professional help has been secured. The newest display, "Careers In Dental Hygiene," features the education of the dental hygienist, locations of schools and the fields of service available to the graduate.

Although records of the 1925 annual session mention "clinics" as well as exhibits, probably they were all exhibits as defined by present standards. A single table clinic, with no title, is listed in the annual meeting program of 1931. Bona fide table clinics were given during the 1933 meeting, perhaps even earlier. Topics were selected by the Clinics Committee and assigned to constituents to present through a chosen member. For many years the ADHA has been invited to present an afternoon of table clinics in conjunction with the ADA clinics. The number is usually limited and, although the best constituent clinics are selected, the ADA reserves the right to make the final choice.

In 1938 the annual session was held in Missouri, which at that time did not allow the practice of dental hygiene. It was through the efforts of R. R. Rhodes, president of the State Board of Dental Examiners, now an honorary member of the ADHA, that the Association was granted permission to demonstrate prophylactic treatments and toothbrushing.

For many years prizes were given for the best clinics. The 1957 Committee on Clinics recommended that the custom be discontinued in that "on awarding gifts that some of the professional aspects of the table clinics was lost. Also, that it was very difficult to know just what articles should be presented as prizes."* Certificates of Appreciation are currently being awarded clinicians.

ADHA Seal, Pin, Oath

The ADA granted permission to use the dental caduceus from their seal as the basis for the ADHA seal designed by Catherine Morris Haas of Bridgeport, Connecticut, in 1928. Until recently official stationery carried this seal and it is engraved on plaques given past presidents, life and hon-

* Minutes of the ADHA, 1923-1971.

orary members. An Association pin designed by Clayton Rudd, D.D.S., under the direction of Ione Jackson of Minnesota, was accepted in 1931. The pin was 14-karat gold, bordered with ten half pearls. The emblem was in dull gold on a black onyx background with the word "Service" in white gold. Guards were available in any special design that a state organization chose to distinguish it from other states. The die has since been lost by the manufacturer and pins are no longer available. A new pin, based on the new Association logo, was designed in 1972. This official pin with the addition of a chip diamond and appropriate engraving is presented to each past president.

As the 25th year of organizational life was celebrated, Frank Lamons, an honorary member from Georgia, assisted in writing an oath for dental hygienists.

Liaison with ADA

From the very beginning a fine working relationship was established with the American Dental Association. In fact, dentists responded more quickly to dental hygienists' requests for the formation of an organization than was anticipated and encouragement and assistance have been continuous. The ADHA has participated with the Dental Association in programs, exhibits, and table clinics. ADHA members have worked with agencies of the ADA in establishing minimum standards of education for dental hygienists, the accreditation program and National Board examinations. Liaison committees have worked cooperatively with the American Association of Dental Examiners and the ADA Councils on Dental Health, Public Relations and Journalism. ADHA members are used as consultants to the ADA Council on Dental Education and as members of accreditation teams. In response to changing times and pressures a Commission on Accreditation of Dental and Dental Auxiliary Programs was established by the 1973 ADA House of Delegates. Two dental hygienists represent the profession on this Commission, one on accreditation proceedings and one on the appeal board.

Before all states provided laws governing dental hygiene practice, the ADA urged states not licensing dental hygienists to do so. The ADA has sponsored several conferences on curricula for dental hygiene programs and functions of dental hygienists. Today representatives from the American Dental Hygienists' Association, American Dental Assistants Association, American Association of Dental Examiners, American Association of Dental Schools and the ADA Council on Dental Education encourage experimentation in the extension of duties of the dental hygienist.

Annual Sessions

The use of a professional parliamentarian was first mentioned in 1930 to assist governing discussions of lengthy and heated matters. For a number of years a parliamentarian was selected from the site of the annual meeting but in 1958 the then District IX recommended that a parliamentarian be secured on an annual basis to be available for consultation as needed during the year as well as at the annual session.

Minutes were first compiled by a dental hygienist secretary but, as they became more involved, a stenographic reporter was hired, and soon it was arranged to have verbatim minutes of both Board and House of Delegates meetings.

A House of Delegates has always been the policy-making body of the Association. Apparently general members were not allowed to attend for the records show that in 1932 the Board voted to allow general members to sit and listen to House of Delegates proceedings.

At first constituent reports were given from the floor; later, written reports were submitted by delegates to be exchanged. Committee reports read and discussed by the Board were re-read along with the Board's comments at the following House of Delegates meeting. Gradually these reports became longer and some facts were misunderstood or lost. Secretary Rebekah Fisk suggested that committee reports be printed and circulated before the meeting to delegates, alternate delegates and state presidents, officers and trustees, to allow more time for discussion. This procedure was so successful that before long trustee reports were included along with the minutes of meetings and summaries of actions taken. Another time-saving device, and a democratic one, was the formation of reference committees to allow informal discussion by the general membership before the House of Delegates met for formal action on resolutions.

War years brought many restrictions to citizens and dental hygienists were no exception. The 1942 annual session was cancelled when the national emergency made travel almost impossible, so at the last minute scientific session plans had to be dropped and all business conducted by mail. Three years later, when restrictions again prevented a general meeting, the Board appointed an Ad Interim Committee to meet and conduct necessary business. This was such a successful way of handling certain portions of business that the Ad Interim Committee came to be an established committee of the Board. It was composed of the president, president elect, secretary, treasurer and three trustees.

The Ad Interim Committee of war years functioned as a standing committee of the Association for thirteen years, meeting in Chicago during the ADA Mid-Winter Meeting because many dental hygienists were already in attendance. By 1955 there was discussion of the Ad Interim Committee meeting becoming a full Board meeting, but no action was taken. The increase in business to be considered demanded another change, that the Board meet two days before the annual session rather than conduct its business during the session. 1958 marked the first Midyear Board meeting.

Employment and Practice Problems

War time also created changes in emphasis. Dental hygienists were urged to join the Red Cross and be active in its programs and to work with the armed services. The United States Army established many positions for dental hygienists in the various camps and army centers throughout the country and legislative action was undertaken by the Association to try to include these dental hygienists in the lists of commissioned officers. One issue of the *Journal* contained excerpts from letters of a dental hygienist who was a "Doughnut Girl" with the Red Cross in France.

President Frances Stoll was appointed in 1949 by the Veterans' Bureau of the United States as Consultant in Dental Hygiene to the Assistant Medical Director. Her assignment was to survey Veterans' Hospitals for potential need for dental hygienists and to recommend the number of dental hygienists needed. Her report recommended that the Civil Service classification of dental hygienists be raised from sub-professional (SP3 and SP4) to professional (P1 and P2) ratings.

Establishing a national employment bureau with a registrar in each state association to funnel information to a central clearing agency was an Association attempt to aid dentists treating the civilian population. Lack of information, understanding and communication kept this endeavor from achieving results and it was discarded after a few years. Although an employment bureau was not feasible on a national level, it was recommended as a suitable activity of state or local groups.

Since many national activities were curtailed it was suggested that attention should be given to strengthening constituent associations. At the suggestion of the chairman of the ADA Civil Defense Committee, ADHA formed a similar committee which was active until the need was outgrown.

Administration

The Bylaws outline the basic duties of officers but their many responsibilities and obligations had never been accurately outlined and certainly not reevaluated. In July of 1958, following the first Mid-Year Board Meeting, an Officer's Conference was held and these items were discussed. More recently, in 1970, a Trustee's Workshop was held to outline duties, responsibilities and functions of the trustees and their relationships with Central Office constituents, components and other trustees. ADHA presidents traditionally have been leaders and have made many far-reaching recommendations. Board members, too, have suggested innovative changes for the betterment of the Association and its individual members.

Continual growth of an organization requires its members to pause from time to time and review its structure and function so that it may better meet its stated objectives and the needs of its membership. With this in mind in 1941 the president-elect, Mrs. Isabel Kendrick, was appointed chairman of a committee to survey reorganization of the Association. Each year the secretary commented on an increasing work load which made it impossible for her to practice dental hygiene full time and fulfill her duties as a volunteer officer. The report stated that it was imperative that a central office be established. What was considered to be the biggest step in the development of the ADHA was taken in 1948 when the office of executive secretary was created as a part-time position with a salary. Duties of the secretary and treasurer were reapportioned and duties of business manager of the *Journal* were added to the secretary's new position. Rebekah Fisk, who had been secretary for several years, was appointed by the Board as the first paid secretary of the Association. One year later Miss Fisk resigned in order to accept a dental hygiene teaching position and was replaced by Margaret E. Swanson. As benefits accrued from the services of the executive secretary it became obvious in 1953 that, to maintain increased membership services, the office should become a full-time, paid position. Miss Swanson accepted and continued in that position until she resigned in 1967. John S. LoSasso, not a dental hygienist but trained in business, was appointed executive director of the Association in 1968 by the Board, followed by Carl H. Hauber, C.A.E. in 1971.

A committee appointed to study the needs of Central Office, including five-year long-range plans, reported their recommendations at the 1957 meeting. Their report included the need for a full-time executive secretary with a salary and the recommendation that Central Office be moved from Washington, D.C. to Chicago. With such major changes it was suggested that an agency skilled in management studies be employed to help reorganize the Association so that there would be impartial, efficient business management, and to revise the Constitution and Bylaws to conform to current Association practices. The cost of such service and the availability of funds were questioned by delegates who requested the committee to obtain cost estimates before taking further action. A pre-survey committee was appointed to make this determination.

A business management firm was employed in 1965 by the Association to develop a prospectus for implementing the activities of the ADHA committees, officers and Central Office. Parts of the report were accepted and implemented while further recommendations were made. As an outgrowth of this activity an Operations and Procedures Manual was developed, and a Long Range Planning Committee in conjunction with committee chairmen produced a report which included the major and specific goals for Association administration, Committees on Dental Health, Dental Hygiene Education, Membership, Legislation, Publications, Public Relations, Finance, Dental Hygiene Practice, the Board of Trustees and the House of Delegates.

As predicted when Central Office was moved to Chicago, proximity to the Dental Association became an advantage and rental costs were offset by savings in travel expenses. As staff members were employed and more work and storage space were needed, larger quarters were leased in the new ADA building.

Communications

A Newsletter was urgently requested by the membership. Since it was costly to produce and mail it was proposed that more information be included in the *Journal* and better communication be established among trustees. Members were persistent and, after the establishment of a Newsletter for Board members and constituent and component presidents, it was agreed that it would be made available upon request. Requests were so numerous that the Newsletter is now distributed regularly to each member.

From time to time discussion centered around a motion picture depicting dental hygiene. Should it be directed to dental health education of the general public, or should it encourage the dental profession to utilize dental hygienists? And should the Association seek a grant or fund the project from its reserve fund? The result of these deliberations was a recruitment film, "A Bright Future," funded by the Association in order that supervision and content would rest solely with the Association. A series of lantern slides was developed from this film. Both media are available for purchase or loan. "A Bright Future" has been shown at career-day programs and organizational meetings, and has been promoted through television screening.

International Relations

The Association has been active in the field of international relations. Correspondence with schools and associations of foreign countries has promoted the exchange of information. At the request of European dentists American dental hygienists have practiced in Switzerland and Holland to demonstrate the capabilities of dental hygienists to provide the benefits of dental hygiene practice to the dentist and his patients. American dental hygienists have been and are assisting in establishing dental hygiene educational programs in Europe.

The World Health Organization employs an American dental hygienist as Technical Officer; her duties include collection, tabulation and preliminary analysis of WHO information related to current program activities of the Dental Health Unit, preparation of scientific papers, reports and correspondence concerning technical matters in dental health. WHO provides consultant services for countries wishing to establish dental hygiene or dental auxiliary programs.*

Canada and the United States have close relationships in educational programs and associations. The first school for dental hygienists in Canada

* Myers, S. E.: WHO and dental auxiliaries around the world. JADHA, 4:32, 1970.

at the University of Toronto was opened in 1951 and six schools are now in operation at the University of Alberta, University of British Columbia, the University of Manitoba, Dalhousie University, the University of Toronto and the Universite de Montreal.

The XIII International Dental Congress invited the ADHA to participate in its program in Cologne, Germany, in 1962; President Ragsdale and Executive Secretary Swanson were appointed as official representatives to this meeting. Several members attended and presented table clinics.

The First International Symposium on Dental Hygiene was sponsored by the Association in 1970. Dentists and dental hygienists from the United States, England, The Netherlands and Switzerland presented papers and Italian dentists welcomed the group to Italy. The Second Symposium took participants to Switzerland, the third to England where they again heard dentists and dental hygienists from the United States and other countries. The Fourth Symposium in the Netherlands featured dental hygienists, expanded function auxiliaries and consumer representatives.

Structure and Function

Objectives

The objectives of the American Dental Hygienists' Association as stated in the Constitution are "to cultivate, promote and sustain the art and science of dental hygiene, to represent and safeguard the common interest of the members of the dental hygiene profession, and to contribute toward the improvement of the health of the public."

Constitution and Bylaws

The Association is governed by its Constitution and Bylaws which set the administrative pattern. These are written laws which may be revised or amended from time to time as circumstances dictate, but only by the House of Delegates. The Constitution describes the objectives of the Association, the composition of its membership, its organization, its governing body, officers and meetings. It also tells how it may be amended and closes with a supremacy clause. The Bylaws are detailed rules for governing the Association. The Principles of Ethics are guides to the moral and personal obligations of each member to the profession and public. Incorporation as a non-profit organization (1927) protects the property of the Association, gives exclusive right to its name, and protects its members.

Membership

There are seven classifications for membership. An *Active* Member must be an ethical dental hygienist who has a certificate or degree in dental hygiene granted by an accredited school of dental hygiene (with certain

5a

exceptions) and must belong to constituent and component associations, if such exist. The President of the Association automatically becomes a *Life* Member at the expiration of term of office, and in addition a member in good standing who has made an outstanding contribution to the Association and dental hygiene may be elected by unanimous vote of the Board and a majority vote of the House. An *Associate* Member is an ethical dental hygienist who is practicing dental hygiene in a country other than the United States or its territories under a current license and membership in a national dental hygiene organization, if either or both exist, in the country where the member practices. An *Allied* Member is an individual who is not qualified for Active or Life Membership who supports the goals and objectives of the Association and has been recommended by a Constituent. *Junior* Members are full-time students either undergraduate or working toward a baccalaureate or graduate degree. An *Honorary* Member is an individual, not a dental hygienist, who has gained recognition for contributions to the national or international scope of the art and science of dental hygiene or dental health for an extended period of time, by unanimous vote of the Board and a majority vote of the House may be elected as an Honorary Member. *Retired* Members must have been Active Members either for a period of twenty-five accumulative years, twenty consecutive years, or continuously since date of eligibility for Active Membership and who has either reached the age of at least sixty-two years or, because of disability has retired from practice at an earlier age, and has been recommended by a Constituent.

Benefits of membership in the American Dental Hygienists' Association are professional affiliation to contribute to and direct the growth of the profession. All members receive official publications which contain pertinent scientific material and current activities of the Association. All members may participate at any level in scientific sessions, table clinic programs, seminars and insurance programs. Organized in democratic manner, sound policies have been established and are changed as necessary to advance Association objectives.

House of Delegates

The House of Delegates is the supreme authoritative body of the Association, having all legislative and policy determining powers. It also has various duties imposed by the Bylaws, electing officers and adopting a budget. By resolution, approving or disapproving proposed committee and Board activities, it directs annual activities. The speaker of the House presides at all sessions of the House of Delegates which is composed of the officially certified delegates of the constituents elected according to the Bylaws. The House of Delegates meets once a year to enact the necessary business of the Association. The executive director serves as the secretary of the House.

Board of Trustees

The Board is composed of the elective officers, except the speaker of the House, the twelve trustees and the immediate past president. The appointive officers, the executive director and the director of publications, are ex-officio members of the Board without a vote. The Board meets three times a year, and special meetings can be called. It maintains and supervises the Central Office and all property of the Association, appoints the executive director, director of publications, fills vacancies in appointive or elective offices, bonds officers or employees entrusted with Association funds, appoints committees, reviews reports and makes recommendations to and reports all of its activities to the House.

Officers

Elective officers of the Association are president, president elect, first vice president, second vice president, treasurer and speaker of the House. The president, president elect and vice presidents hold office for one year, or until their successors are installed, and the treasurer and speaker of the House are elected for two-year terms. Appointive officers are the executive director, director of publications, and others as may be required. The duties of the officers are outlined in the Bylaws and are detailed in the Operations and Procedures Manual. The executive director is the executive officer of the Association and carries out policies and programs which have been approved. As head of the Association's Central Office these duties include supervising and coordinating activities of committees and preparation of reports. The executive director is employed by the Board and is accountable to it. The director of publications has full editorial control over the *Journal* and is responsible to the Board. The Association Central Office is in Chicago, under the general supervision of the Board but directly administered by the executive director.

Committees

Committees of the Association are unlimited in number in order to keep pace with the changing needs of dental hygiene activity so necessary to attainment of Association objectives. Committees report to the Board at its mid-year meeting and at the annual session, proposing programs or expressing viewpoints. A great portion of Association work is done by committees, although the Division of Educational Services and the Washington Office are now taking over many administrative responsibilities in areas of education and legislation. Committees recommend policies and all Association members are eligible for appointment. Committees are composed of at least three members appointed for a term of no less than one year with tenure limited to four consecutive years.

The Committee on Community Dental Health studies problems dealing with the improvement of health of the public; cooperates with the ADA and supports its programs; assists constituent and components and other agencies.

The Committee on Dental Hygiene Education is concerned with the improvement of dental hygiene education; upholds standards of education; works with the ADA Council on Dental Education; assists in recruitment of students.

The Committee on Legislation and the Washington representative assist constituents with problems in protecting and furthering the interests of the public and dental hygienists through appropriate activities. Anything affecting public health and the practice of dental hygiene is within their purview.

The Committee on Membership plans and promotes programs to increase membership. A Sub-Committee on Junior Membership is assigned the same responsibilities for encouraging membership of undergraduate dental hygiene students.

The Committee on Scholarship, newly renamed the Committee on Student Financial Aid, manages the scholarship program, develops policies and procedures for awarding scholarships and selects recipients from the applications submitted. Scholarship funds come from the Educational Trust Fund, the American Fund for Dental Health and specially designated grants. Other committees and their duties are defined in the Scopes Manual which is updated at each Board meeting.

Annual Sessions

The Annual Session includes meetings of the House of Delegates, the Board, and reference committees, and scientific presentations and discussions of subjects pertaining to the art and science of dental hygiene and related fields. Admission is limited to members and registered guests.

Educational Trust Fund

The Educational Trust Fund, established on February 3, 1957, is separate from other funds of the Association. Its purpose is "to advance the art and science of dental hygiene; promote public welfare through the development of higher standards of practice in the field of dental hygiene; to encourage and engage in professional education and scientific research in dental hygiene and aid in the health education of the public with respect thereto; to conduct and carry on programs of testing students for achievement and prospective students for aptitude to determine their potentials in the field of dental hygiene and making available the findings and results of such tests to those interested in dental hygiene education; to provide financial assistance at the discretion of the trustees of the fund through scholarships or otherwise to needy, worthy and qualified graduate and undergraduate students of dental hygiene upon such terms and conditions as the trustees of the Fund may determine."* All activities above are exclusively for charitable, scientific, literary or educational purposes. The trustees of the Fund are the president, president elect, treasurer and the executive director as an ex-officio trustee.

Division of Educational Services

The Division of Educational Services functions under the general supervision of the executive director. It is responsible for the continued improvement and development of dental hygiene education programs and the establishment of standards of quality and acceptability for dental hygiene and works closely with the Committees on Dental Hygiene Education, Scholarship and Legislation.

Membership

The Association represents organized dental hygiene, expressing the opinions and wishes of the members. In order to be a valid spokesman for the profession, it needs to represent a majority of active practicing and retired dental hygienists.

Pioneer dentists who recognized benefits to their patients and practices through use of the services of the dental hygienist were most enthusiastic. In contrast, there was active opposition to the dental hygiene movement by dentists in some areas and the passive indifference of others slowed the progress of dental hygiene. Forty-six dental hygienists registered for the 1923 meeting which marked the beginning of a national association for the profession of dental hygiene. Although state associations were represented officially by delegates, membership in the new group was neither automatic nor mandatory. There seems to be no precise record of the number of members the first year, but the president's message of 1927 stated that membership consisted of "about 100 of the 1100 dental hygienists then in the United States." When the second annual meeting was called to order there were 153 recorded members.

The fact that dental organizations and schools were well established and had accessible lines of communication plus the groundwork laid by Dr. Fones no doubt encouraged the acceptance of dental hygiene more quickly by northeastern dentists than by those in other parts of the United States. With 2,000 graduate dental hygienists by 1928, and eighteen constituent associations, membership in the ADHA indicated representation of approximately one quarter of the profession.

The growing numbers of practicing dental hygienists continued to band into new constituent groups to exchange professional information. New membership provisions and classifications added to the Bylaws encouraged growth and, although records of 1933 show twenty-four constituent asso-

* Bylaws, ADHA, 1970.

ciations, there had been an overall loss of ten members—a situation which has never been repeated.

The first effort to increase membership nationally resulted in an increase to 2,613 members in 1949. In following years the Committee on Membership and the Committee on Junior Membership, either separately or as a joint committee, have written to students and graduates encouraging membership in the Association. Questionnaires have been sent to special categories of dental hygienists to try to determine why they did not join the Association or why they dropped membership. Appropriate changes in recruitment approaches are made periodically to increase membership.

Constituent members surveyed non-members individually in 1962 and a campaign, "Project Tomorrow," was conducted by a recruitment agency in 1969-1970. Increasing student involvement is viewed as a major means of encouraging membership in the ADHA but other means of increasing membership will be studied until strong majority representation is achieved.

Junior Membership

The ADA studied the value of offering dental students junior membership in their Association, and in the following year ADHA considered such a classification for their Association. Twelve of the fifteen dental hygiene programs surveyed approved the idea if dues were not more than $1.00. The chairman of the special committee said the Association must offer something "stimulating and valuable" to these students in exchange for dues. When the new membership classification was accepted in 1938 dues were at $1.00, 75¢ of which was for an annual *Journal* subscription. Within three years, eight of the seventeen schools had junior members; today all schools have junior members. A meeting of junior members was held in 1960 at the ADHA annual session. A model Constitution and By-laws were drafted as a guide for individual organizations. By 1966 regional meetings were being held by students, and in 1970 the first state association of junior members was formed in Pennsylvania.

In an attempt to hold junior members' interest in membership, courtesy membership is extended until the end of the year after graduation and they are allowed to participate actively in their constituent and component groups. The ADHA Committee on Membership initiated the use of a student member with full committee privileges in 1970-1971. Under the direction of the Committee on Membership junior members now plan and participate in their own meeting during the ADHA annual session.

Membership Categories

The original Bylaws contained the following classifications: (A) Corporate membership: regularly elected and qualified members of the House of Delegates, (B) General membership: members of constituent societies and others as may be elected or appointed. From time to time these have been amended or altered, adding categories including self-limiting "grand-father" clauses which allowed those few remaining dental hygienists without formal training to become members. In 1974 membership classifications included: Active Members, Life Members, Allied Members, Associate Members, Junior Members, Honorary Members, Retired Members. These are defined on page 121.

Exclusion from membership through race, color or creed has never been incorporated in ADHA Bylaws, but through use of the word "female" male dental hygienists were excluded until 1964. The first man was licensed as a dental hygienist in Oregon, and in 1970 there were three recent gradu-ates and ten male students enrolled in educational programs. In 1957 the Association's open membership policy was affirmed and constituents were requested to review their Bylaws and revise them to conform with those of the parent association.

Finances

A professional association exists in part to safeguard the interests of its members and to offer them services which will encourage interest and participation in the organization. Mundane as money may be, no profes-sional organization can operate without financial support.

The American Dental Hygienists' Association was founded without a treasury. In two years, when the 1925 general meeting was held, dues in the amount of $128.20 had been collected and the Fones Alumni Associa-tion had donated $50.00. Expenses of the two-year period were $62.95, leaving a balance of $115.25 with which to start another year. After fifty years of operation, the budget, both income and expenses, exceed $500,000.

Dues

Dues originally were $2.00 but they were increased to $3.00 to include the *Journal* subscription. Dues raises have been infrequent, a real tribute to those who watched expenses carefully and to those who spent their own funds for travel on Association business. When the second dues raise was discussed in 1946 it was recognized that compared to other volunteer or-ganizations and compared to unions, dental hygienists pay very low dues, a fact which is still true. With minor dissent the dues were raised to $5.00. As general expenses increased and an attempt was made to reimburse offi-cers and trustees partially for out-of-pocket expenses, another dues raise, this time to $7.00, was necessary in 1954.

Several years of discussion took place before the increase to the sum of $15.00 was accepted in January, 1961. The necessity of underwriting the Division of Educational Services and other vitally needed ADHA pro-grams, the desire to institute more membership service programs in areas of legislation and communication, and the need for expanding the staff to administer these programs properly directed the 1971 dues increase to

$25.00. When ADHA membership services and dues are compared to those offered by comparable organizations, the cost is still negligible. Junior members' dues have escalated from $1.00 to $2.00, then in 1971 to $3.00, primarily due to increased *Journal* costs. A registration fee at the annual session has been in effect for several years and the 1974 House of Delegates voted a dues increase to become effective in 1976.

Budget

The growing income and expenditures of the Association necessitated appointment of a budget committee, and the first genuine "budget" was presented by the committee chairman, Margaret Swanson, in 1949. As reference committees of the Board evolved, a finance committee comprised of three trustees and the treasurer was formed. This committee is the Reference Committee on Budget for the House of Delegates. An accounting firm is employed to recommend efficient bookkeeping procedures and to make regular audits of all accounts.

Journal

A common interest is the foundation of any organization. To sustain interest and remain a practical functioning entity, there must be constant satisfactory accomplishment of these goals. Communication is essential for any organization, for it binds its members together, reinforcing and cementing their objectives.

Distances were great, travel was difficult and money was scarce in the 1920's, so attendance at meetings was small although membership and representation grew. As an aid to fulfillment of Association objectives, to establish and maintain effective communications between the Association and its members, and to aid in educating the public toward dental hygiene and dental health, the *Journal of The American Dental Hygienists' Association* was established and published monthly starting in January of 1927, edited by Dorothy Bryant.

At the invitation of the Dental Association, delegates of the second annual meeting of the ADHA appointed an editorial committee to prepare oral health instructional material for the Department of Dental Health of the ADA *Journal.*

Inexperienced as they were, the early leaders of the ADHA recognized that without communication the viability of the organization would be lost. The American Dental Laboratory Association offered space in their publication but the Board decided to establish a new professional journal, for a professional journal is a mechanism for both public and professional relations. A separate fund was established for this project, its money to be a portion of membership dues supplemented by advertising income and other subscription fees, which were $1.00 a year.

The sixteen pages of Volume I, No. 1, published on schedule, included the president's address from the 1926 annual meeting, an article by the current president, an article on membership, a report of the Philadelphia meeting, "A Word About Finances," an editorial and a delegate's report of the Michigan State Dental Hygienists' Association meeting. Nutrition lectures at Forsyth were announced and New York State dental hygienists welcomed the first issue of the *Journal*. At the end of the first year of publication the report showed that the *Journal* had served Association membership admirably, but its financial position was unfavorable. This was not particularly alarming for the first efforts of a small non-profit group but steps were outlined to improve the situation.

The *Journal* editor requested appointment of an advertising manager who could devote time to securing more advertising so that the publication could earn its own way. Since the *Journal* was financially separate from the Association, a loan was requested from it so that this membership service might be continued. Subscription fees were added to dues in 1928, making them a total of $3.00.

The following year Dorothy Bryant resigned and Margaret Jeffreys undertook editorial duties. The *Journal* was still having monetary problems but it was growing in stature and circulation. Mildred Gilsdorf was appointed as chairman of reporters and a state reporter was appointed from each constituent association. Leading dentists and dental hygienists contributed scientific articles; historical and inspirational articles were included; practical hints were exchanged through a question-and-answer column; annual reports and a summary of the annual session routinely were included.

The *Journal's* financial status continued to deteriorate during the depression years in spite of all efforts and it was suggested that it be issued on a bi-monthly or quarterly basis until it achieved solvency. As a result, the *Journal* became a quarterly publication in 1934. In conformity with other professional journals an advertising code was adopted and is still followed. The difficulty of finding reporters for each state led to asking each constituent president to assume this responsibility. District trustees currently collect material from their constituents and submit it to the *Journal* for publication.

The first ten years were years of learning, frustrations and rewards. The editor, Margaret Jeffreys, reported that the *Journal* had survived and seemed to be recovering, and recommended that it be published on a monthly basis as soon as possible. That was in 1937. In 1970 it still was issued quarterly but it became a bi-monthly publication in 1971 and will be produced monthly in the near future.

When Margaret Jeffreys resigned, Chief Reporter Mary Owen assumed editorship. The next change was seven years later when Shirley Ellis held the position for two years, followed by Rebekah Fisk, interim editor for one issue until the appointment of Isabell Kendrick. Three years later, in 1952, Belle Fiedler became editor and acted in that capacity successfully for nine years. During her years as editor she was elected president of the American Association of Dental Editors, and, in appreciation of her contribution to the Association through the *Journal,* she was elected to honorary membership on retirement. In 1970, under new Bylaws provisions, this was rescinded and she was elected to life membership.

World War II changed the *Journal* as well as personal lives. When the Office of Price Administration in 1941 asked for conservation of paper, ADHA responded by voting to limit the journal content to 40 pages and to mail it without a wrapper. Some members said it was unthinkable to mail it "naked," but it was sent thus for the duration. "Postage Guaranteed" was put on each copy so undeliverable copies would be returned instead of being destroyed, and two-year-old engraved metal plates used in printing the *Journal* were turned in to the government for scrap. When war restrictions were removed, the finances of the *Journal* were in a healthier state and it seemed time for a change. In the early 1950's the cover of the *Journal* was redesigned by artist Harold Stoll, husband of Past President Frances Stoll.

"Women Only" a controversial editorial written in 1954 urged the exclusion of males from dental hygiene. Protests were registered but it was the decision of the Board that it was the editor's prerogative to express an opinion and to stimulate the thinking of the membership.

Annual reports of committees and of the annual session customarily were printed in the *Journal* but inclusion became more difficult as activities increased and reports grew longer. The 1956 Board decided to discontinue printing such committee reports and to mail them separately but to continue to print a summary of the annual meeting.

The first *Journal* staff conference was held in 1960 to review current procedures and establish future goals. At that time it was decided to increase the scientific content of the *Journal* and to publicize available postgraduate courses. Although members wanted a Central Office Newsletter this was not feasible financially, so the Central Office Section in the *Journal* was expanded. When the Newsletter became a reality this section was dropped from the *Journal.*

The House of Delegates approved a new name for the *Journal* in 1972 and it is now known as DENTAL HYGIENE, the Journal of the American Dental Hygienists' Association. It became a monthly publication in January 1975 and will again incorporate the Central Office newsletter, Newsbriefs.

With Miss Fieldler's resignation Lucille Klein was appointed, followed six years later by D. Jeanne Bedore Collins. When Mrs. Collins resigned in March, 1970, the Board appointed Mrs. Wilma Motley as editor.

Each year since 1967 the *Journal* staff has conducted workshops for constituent and component editors during annual sessions to assist them in their editorial duties.

Officers

Association Bylaws provide that officers serve for one year or until their successors are elected and installed. Because there were no general meetings in 1924, 1942 and 1945 there could be no elections; therefore those incumbent presidents, Mrs. Winifred Hart, Mrs. Mary Zoepfel and Margaret Jeffreys, each automatically served two terms. Officers of the Association include a president elect who becomes president at the next election, practically precluding the possibility of a president running for a second term. Only once has a president elect been unable to serve, thus making election of a president for the ensuing year mandatory. Margaret Ryan resigned as president elect to become the first ADHA Director of the Division of Educational Services in 1967. President Wilma Motley ran for a second term of office and became the only president elected to serve twice.

Reimbursement of Expenses

The first officers were volunteers who paid their own personal expenses connected with Association activities. It did not take long to recognize that the secretary worked a great many hours for the Association and she was granted $50.00 per year as an honorarium. The same year the Board gave the treasurer an honorarium. The next step ahead was paying rail fare, Pullman accommodations, hotel room and ticket to the official banquet of the annual session for the president, and the following year for the secretary.

After sixteen years of personal expense and devoted service, serious consideration was made of reimbursement for Board members' expenses. The sum of $5.00 each for attendance at a meeting was proposed and rejected in 1939. The next year it was proposed that hotel accommodations be paid for the Board during the annual session but the motion received no second. The secretary's salary was doubled and the treasurer became responsible for collecting dues. Again, reimbursement for officers was promoted and this time is was agreed that the president, secretary and treasurer receive $25.00 for convention expenses in addition to travel benefits, and that the rest of the official family receive hotel expenses at $3.00 a day plus conference breakfast and official tea and banquet tickets "if they were used."

The president, not reimbursed for travel by the Association, could not attend many constituent meetings, but as the need for national representation was recognized the president or her official designate were authorized to travel at Association expense if national interest were involved; otherwise the constituent should pay for the visit. Soon the president, president elect, and vice presidents received $50.00 for partial reimbursement of expenses. Financial aid for officers was discussed officially again several years later when air coach fare and $15.00 per diem for official ADHA Board and annual session meetings were allowed. The per diem was increased to

$30.00 to adjust for inflation in 1969. The same reimbursement is budgeted for committees who meet officially. With the creation of the office of executive secretary, the salary was made commensurate with the new responsibilities; as the office became a full-time position the salary was increased accordingly. As of 1971 district trustees are financed by the Association to attend each of their constituents' meetings once; other district expenses are underwritten by the district membership.

Bylaws

A Constitution and Bylaws were presented to the 1923 organizational meeting. These documents were accepted provisionally so officers could be elected, but it was stipulated that a committee be appointed to make suggested changes. The committee completed its work and the Constitution and Bylaws were adopted formally in 1925.

Bylaws are operating rules and, as such, must be sufficiently flexible that programs can be operated or administered effectively with the least amount of delay. If Bylaws are restrictive, frequent amendments must be made; if they are permissive, stated in broad terms with detailed procedures outlined, the document is easier to change and fewer amendments are necessary to operate the organization. As needs have changed Association Bylaws have been amended, but there have been few complete revisions at approximate intervals of ten years. Association structure changed recently and Bylaws are being amended to conform with the mandates of the House of Delegates.

Almost from the beginning the ADHA urged state associations to revise their Bylaws to conform with national Bylaws, and some years much attention was directed to this. In 1950 a supremacy clause was added which provided that the ADHA Constitution and Bylaws "shall be the supreme law of this organization and all its constituents and they shall be bound thereby."*
The following year it was reported that all state Constitutions and Bylaws were in conformity with those of the parent association.

Membership

Some of the first Bylaws changes related to membership. In 1920 only six states licensed dental hygienists. Eighteen years later 38 states and the territory of Hawaii had provided legally for the practice of dental hygiene, and by 1951 all states licensed the dental hygienist. A list of states and dates of first licensure of dental hygienists is included in the Appendix.

Membership requirements have been modified to accommodate situations as they arose. The Legislative Committee believed that a dental hygienist, regardless of color, was entitled to ADHA membership. However,

* Bylaws, ADHA, 1970.

some states' membership requirements automatically excluded blacks. Many years elapsed before all restrictions were removed and, in the meantime, the National Dental Hygienists' Association was organized in the 1940's by and for black dental hygienists and functioned approximately three years. In the spring of 1962 all the black dental hygienists known to faculty members of Meharry Medical College, Nashville, Tennessee, were contacted and invited to meet in Detroit at the time of the National Dental Association meeting for the purpose of reactivating the organization. Twelve dental hygienists met, elected temporary officers and appointed a constitution committee. Black dental hygienists located in each convention city were encouraged to organize and provide a forum where mutual concerns could be discussed. The activities of the group were generally limited to the preparation of the scientific and social programs for the annual meeting. Many NDHA members hold dual membership in ADHA.*

There were no membership provisions for preceptor trained (apprentice rather than formally educated and trained) dental hygienists. Dental associations in Kansas would not recognize the dental hygiene association unless these dental hygienists were allowed to join. The Georgia State Board of Dental Examiners ruled that anyone who had had two years of experience as a dental assistant and had been recommended by her employer, regardless of the lack of formal training in an accredited school, could be licensed to practice dental hygiene in that state. In Texas the state dental association refused to recognize the dental hygienists' association unless a clause was inserted limiting the membership to members of the Caucasian race. Special consideration was given to Texas non-graduate dental hygienists who received a certificate from special courses given by Baylor University College of Dentistry for "grandmother" dental hygienists, provided that ADA accredited the program. Naturally some situations were resolved more easily than others but, eventually, and with help from the ADA, compromises were reached. A "grandfather clause" with an expiration date was inserted in the ADHA Bylaws and restrictions for race, color or creed were specifically prohibited by the Constitution and Bylaws.

Another major change in the Bylaws was the elimination of the word "female" in 1964, thereby admitting males to membership.

Board of Trustees

Originally the elected officers were not allowed to vote in Board sessions. Too often there were not enough trustees present to reach a quorum to conduct its business and, as a result, officers were allowed to vote. Bylaws were amended to legalize this procedure and the entire Board the right to vote in the House of Delegates rather than to continue as ex-officio members of the House without the right to vote. When Bylaws were revised

*Shirley R. Pike, R.D.H., M.P.H., Ann Arbor, Michigan.

in 1968 the trustees once more became ex-officio members of the House without the right to vote.

Speaker of the House of Delegates

As duties of the president became more extensive a speaker of the House of Delegates was suggested. When accepted, a speaker was elected but because of illness could not attend the following annual session. The whole matter was then reconsidered and referred to the Bylaws Committee who tabled the question. Five years later, in 1961, when a Bylaws amendment created the position, Marjorie Thornton, a past president of the Association, was elected and became the first speaker of the House to preside at an annual session.

House of Delegates

Until 1961 each constituent association was allowed one delegate to the annual session. As membership grew it seemed more democratic to have proportional representation and a formula was adopted, allowing each state to have one delegate for up to 100 members, and one delegate for each 100 members over that number. Consideration is being given to limiting the size of the House of Delegates so it will never become unwieldy. If a limit is placed on the total number of delegates, another formula for representation will be arranged for use when the maximum number has been reached.

Principles of Ethics

The first "Principles of Ethics" (p. 20) were stated broadly as were some subsequent revisions, but in 1953 a committee was directed to rewrite these principles defining ethical behavior under as many headings as might be indicated. This detailed code prevailed until 1969 when it once more was rewritten in broad statements. The House of Delegates adopted the newly written Principles of Ethics in 1974 (pp. 20-21). An Association platform, to be reviewed each year by the Board, was also adopted in 1969. The platform (see Appendix) is a declaration of principles designed to promote and insure the excellence of the professional standards of the American Dental Hygienists' Association, strengthen the function of the Association, and assure optimum discharge of its responsibilities.

Trustee Districts

Trustees always have been a part of the governing body of the Association. The first trustees were elected "at large" from the entire membership. As more state organizations were chartered a means of equal representation on the Board was indicated. It was suggested that the United States be divided into nine districts, patterned after those of the ADA. Each district would be represented by a trustee elected from within its membership. This plan was adopted, with the addition of the immediate past president as a member of the Board for one year.

For fifteen years this plan worked well, but once more Association growth dictated changes. This time states were reapportioned into twelve districts. Belief in the trustee's obligation to serve district members through visiting constituent meetings and holding district meetings prompted the latest redistricting in 1970. The number of districts, twelve, remained the same, but states within the district boundaries have been changed making it geographically possible for the trustee to visit and work with each constituent association.

Constituent Associations

Individual states have also experienced problems. Legislative problems have been met individually by the state but supported by the ADHA. The following are "landmark" cases. The distances between major population centers in northern and southern California prompted members to petition the Association for permission to form two constituent associations, represented by one delegate who would alternate between the groups. This was granted but did not provide adequate representation and in a few years ADHA was again petitioned, this time requesting a delegate from each group. Bylaws were quoted to support the request: that under the Chapter on Constituents, Powers and Duties, each constituent has the power to elect from among its members a delegate to the House of Delegates of this Association; and under Privileges, each constituent association shall be represented in the business sessions of this Association by at least one delegate. California is the only state to have two fully qualified and recognized constituent associations. Since that time other states, Washington in 1955, for example, have petitioned on the same basis, but requests have been rejected.

Association Committees

The House of Delegates in 1968 deleted the listing of standing committees of the Association to allow the House to establish committees as needed. Provision was made for inclusion of at least three members, each of whom shall serve for one year with a maximum of four years, one member to be appointed as chairman. All committees are approved by the Board and are budgeted to meet during the year when documented justification is presented. Their duties are directed by the House of Delegates and specified by the Board of Trustees. By direction of the Board each officer is appointed as consultant to a committee or committees.

Legislation

Many times it is assumed that a professional organization approves or disapproves certain legislation, but only an adopted policy statement can be used to give or withhold official support. Because a dentist, an opponent of fluoridation, cited Fones' method of reducing tooth decay, the ADHA was prompted in 1956 to adopt a policy statement supporting fluoridation of public water supplies as a means of reducing tooth decay in children. This policy statement, later reaffirmed, is still used by constituent and component associations as they work toward this public dental health goal. The first extension of services of the dental hygienist, total application of fluorides, was supported by the dental profession and began as early as 1950.

The ADA officially opposed the Foran Bill of 1958 which would have provided health care through federal compulsory medical insurance because it was not in the best interests of the recipients. The ADHA supported the Dental Association stand. More currently, ADHA officially supports federal preventive dentistry programs and opposes preceptorship training of dental hygienists.

The Association routinely has offered advice to constituents when legal problems have arisen but has encouraged the constituent to take the initiative in solving them. Occasionally letters have been written in support of a state association position or a policy statement has been adopted when precedents are being set. In 1956 a dentist was allowed to take the California State Board Dental Hygiene Examination on grounds that the education of a dentist was greater in scope than that of the dental hygienist. The implications of this precedent, and a similar incident in Oregon in 1957, led to changes in requirements for eligibility to take dental hygiene licensure examinations. They now read "graduation from an accredited school of dental hygiene." This requirement is again being challenged by dentists on the same grounds as before.

At the end of World War II the Association's Committee on Legislation was concerned with the possibility of veterans who had been trained by the armed services applying for the dental hygiene licensing examination after return to civilian life. State boards of dental examiners were urged to uphold the educational qualifications for dental hygienists in their states and to refer all service-trained personnel to accepted schools of dental hygiene. Military trained dental auxiliaries are a potential resource for health manpower and consideration currently is being given to means of utilizing their skills in civilian practice.

Civil Service

As early as 1927 the Association became interested in the inadequate recognition of dental hygienists working in departments of public health and government civil service positions. When nurses were trained to perform some dental hygiene procedures the Association protested this use of unqualified personnel. The reason given by the government was that dental hygienists on the list of applicants were not qualified, so the Association drew up a list of necessary qualifications for dental hygienists applying for Civil Service positions and submitted it to the government.

Dental hygienists, patriotically, wanted to offer professional services in the war effort. The ADHA believed that dental hygienists should be given commissions comparable to those of nurses with equal educational background. A request was sent to the Surgeon General; the Military Affairs Committee disapproved it. A bill to commission degree dieticians and physical therapists in the Medical Department of the U.S. Army was heard by the House Committee and Sophie Gurevich (Booth), ADHA Vice President, testified, requesting that dental hygienists be included. This request, too, was refused.

A War Service Committee of the Association was then formed and funds appropriated to be used to try to secure commission status for army dental hygienists. The chairman of the ADA Legislative Committee helped draft a statement. The attempt was unsuccessful but it was instrumental in stimulating provision for appointment or enrollment in the Medical Department of technical and professional female personnel in categories required for duty outside the continental United States by executive order.

Another joint legislative effort of ADA and ADHA was to bring to the attention of the Civil Service Committee and the War Department the need of civilian personnel to be properly qualified to hold positions to which they were appointed. This was because the Army and Navy were giving "short courses" to women who were then permitted to work in the service as "dental hygienists." In 1971 the Army offers commissions as second lieutenants to dental hygienists with a bachelor's degree.

Licensure Laws

Many years ago, in 1948, expansion of the dental hygienist's duties was discussed by the ADA. A special committee was appointed by the ADHA to study and evaluate legislative trends related to functions and responsibilities of the dental hygienist. The Association reaffirmed liaison with appropriate agencies of the dental profession to institute a review of licensure laws relating to the practice of dental hygiene. They agreed that laws that do not detail the dental hygienist's functions better support the efforts of the dental profession to provide preventive dental services. All states have been urged to reword their dental practice acts so that dentists may delegate duties to dental hygienists according to the amendable rules and regulations of the state board of dentistry. Dental hygienists are appointed as consultants by the boards of dentistry in several states and are "expert examiners" for dental hygiene examinations in at least two states.

A definition of dental hygiene practice for use in dental practice acts which provide for delegation of additional functions through rules and regulations was drafted and adopted by the Association in 1968. "Dental hygiene may be practiced only by a licensed dentist or licensed dental hygienist. Dental hygiene practice shall be defined as those clinical procedures which can have a direct effect upon the physical well-being of the patient but do not constitute the practice of dentistry. This shall include: removing all hard and soft deposits and stains; polishing natural and restored surfaces of teeth; polishing restorations; removing excess cement; performing clinical examination of teeth and surrounding tissue for diagnosis by the dentist; and performing other procedures delegated by the dentist in accord with the rules and regulations of the state board of dentistry."

ADHA Washington Representative

Constant surveillance is necessary in order to keep pace with the rapid changes in all health care professions and in their systems of delivery of health services. The ADHA is in a position to monitor and evaluate these changes and keep pace with them. The Association must continue to be aware of proposals throughout the country and must be able to advise wisely, presenting factual material in a manner acceptable to dentistry, legislators and the public. In the interest of the public, the aim must be to express the concern of the profession in all legislative matters and to promote programs that will benefit the public. The Association at national and state levels should be preparing itself to introduce legislation benefitting the public rather than opposing legislation introduced by others.

The need for the Association to keep informed of new developments in legislation, particularly at the federal level, to prepare factual statements and to give testimony before Senate and House committees led to the creation of a new position. Mrs. Diane McCain, a dental hygienist and a past officer of the Association, is the first to be the Association's Washington representative. The primary objective of this office is to provide information to the Association related to federal programs affecting the delivery of health services, and through cooperation with appropriate governmental and private agencies promote public interest in health related programs.*

Responsibilities include liaison activities with members of Congress, Congressional committees, health professions and allied health professions organizations, federal agencies and other appropriate agencies. The delegate also reviews federal legislation and activity of interest to dental hygiene and reports to the Association.*

The Washington representative and an administrative assistant work from an office in the new ADA Washington offices.

Educational Programs

Records of 1930 mention that dental hygienists had participated in Dental Health Week with children for several years. Invited by the Ameri-

* McCain, Diane: Objectives and responsibilities of the Washington office. ADHA, 1970.

can Dental Association to appoint a committee as a liaison group between the two associations, the Council on Dental Health and the ADHA Committee on Dental Health Education discussed National Children's Dental Health Day and plans for promoting dental health throughout the country. As a result a resolution was presented by the ADA and adopted by the United States Senate and House of Representatives designating the first Monday in February as National Children's Dental Health Day. Since then the day has been extended to a week and dental hygienists actively participate in special dental health programs.

Health materials were collected by this committee and listed under the title "Educational Reprints and Materials Available from Various Sources," a list which has been updated periodically. In more recent years "Project Pointers" was developed as a guide for constituent and component organizations in planning and carrying out community dental health programs. There is now a Committee on Community Dental Health to encourage these and other relevant activities.

The responsibilities of the first Dental Hygiene Education Committee included dental health for the public and dental hygienists as well as the education of dental hygienists. Increased activity in both fields soon led to the formation of two separate committees.

Dental Hygiene Schools

Twelve schools of dental hygiene graduated 2,000 dental hygienists by 1928. Twenty years later the number of educational programs had increased, but only to seventeen, and the number of graduates was estimated at 8,000. Of these, some 5,500 to 6,000 were in active practice. The 1965 Survey of Dental Practice stated that 15,400 dental hygienists were employed in the United States. By 1969 the estimated number of employed dental hygienists was 18,000. In early 1974 there were 160 operating programs, 138 of these being two years in length. Twenty-three schools offer both a two and a four year course.

Dental hygienists have always been in demand, but the costs of establishing new programs and the lack of qualified faculty kept establishment of new schools to a minimum.

Formal dental hygiene educational programs progressed from Fones' six-months course to a one-year course of instruction to a two-year course, most of the programs in dental school settings. One school offers a four-year degree course with dental hygiene integrated throughout the four years and others offer bachelor's degrees through a variety of combinations of dental hygiene and pre- or postdental hygiene courses in the arts and sciences. In addition, in 1970 there were three bachelor's degree programs specifically designed for teacher education and four master's degree programs in dental hygiene education.

"Principles of Dental Hygiene Education," approved by the Association, is a series of statements outlining the general philosophy and goals of various types of programs. In summary, Certificate and/or Associate Degree Dental Hygiene Programs should be at an educational level equivalent to at least the first two years of baccalaureate degree education. Curricula should prepare graduates for admission to baccalaureate degree programs and should be designed to prepare dental hygienists to provide preventive and therapeutic dental hygiene services. Graduates should have the potential necessary to assume increased responsibility to perform complete units of clinical practice within the realm of their delegated responsibilities. Curricula may be designed to prepare students to provide additional services as determined by the projected dental health needs; potential for the certificate dental hygienist to provide services to meet those needs; and the ability of the dental hygiene program to provide instruction in these areas.

Baccalaureate Degree Dental Hygiene Programs should provide an education consistent with standards in higher education. The baccalaureate curriculum should be conducted at a level which allows for admission to university graduate programs and should incorporate a substantive body of knowledge in the social, behavioral, and biological sciences prerequisite for entrance into advanced disciplines. These programs should provide advanced knowledge and skills in dental hygiene. The curricula should prepare graduates for expanded roles in the delivery of oral health services. These services shall be determined by projected dental health needs, potential for the dental hygienist to provide services to meet these needs, and the ability of the program to provide instruction in these areas. Graduates should have the educational background necessary for increased responsibility in decision making and in the performance of complete units of clinical practice within the realm of their delegated responsibilities. The curricula should be designed to prepare students not only for preventive and therapeutic dental hygiene services but also to assume positions of additional responsibility and leadership in one or more of the following areas: dental hygiene education; dental public health; hospital dentistry; public and private schools; and research.

Master's Degree Dental Hygiene Programs should be at an educational level equivalent to master's degree programs in other disciplines and will allow further pursuit of advanced degrees. Curricula should be designed to prepare dental hygienists for increased leadership and responsibility in one or more of the following areas: administrative positions and/or consultant positions in public health or other agencies; administrative and/or teaching positions in dental hygiene education programs; research in related fields; increased depth in a basic or dental science; and preparation for the further pursuit of advanced degrees.*

Parent Institutions for Dental Hygiene Programs

The Association has recommended that schools of dental hygiene be established in institutions of higher education which can provide educa-

* Minutes of the ADHA, 1923-1974.

tional resources necessary for developing dental hygiene curricula that will meet accreditation standards, that courses be acceptable for credit toward a bachelor's degree, and that schools not now offering baccalaureate degree courses arrange to do so where possible. The definition of dental hygiene practice has been revised and schools are urged to experiment with extended functions of the dental hygienist. Curriculum changes to include education of dental students to the use of the dental hygienist are also encouraged. The U.S. Public Health Service "Dental TEAM" (Training in Expanded Auxiliary Management) Project implements this concept.

The first programs in technical schools were established in 1948. With the growth of community colleges dental hygiene programs have mushroomed, and in 1974 these accounted for more than half (53 per cent) of dental hygiene programs. Many others are in planning stages.

Scholarships

Each year an increasing number of scholarships become available through the Association, donations of dental hygienists, the American Fund for Dental Health, American Dental Association endowments and dental manufacturers. These are granted to students so that they may finish their dental hygiene training, and to practicing and newly graduated dental hygienists to enable them to obtain baccalaureate or master's degrees.

Most scholarships today are awarded as stipends, based on academic achievement, demonstrated need and potential success of the student, rather than as specified sums of money. The increase in numbers of applicants has made it necessary for a consultant to be utilized in setting criteria for evaluation of applications and for an individual in the Division of Educational Services to be responsible for supervising this activity.

March 15, 1938, marked the death of Alfred Civilion Fones, affectionately known as the Father of Dental Hygiene. At the following annual session a memorial resolution was adopted and a loan fund of $1,000 was established in his name. This is now one of the ADHA scholarships. Another scholarship has been named the Irene Newman Scholarship in honor of his assistant, the first dental hygienist. A bronze plaque memorializing Dr. Fones, cosponsored by the American Dental Hygienists' Association, the Connecticut Dental Hygienists' Association and the Bridgeport Dental Hygienists' Association, was presented to and is displayed in the Fones School of Dental Hygiene, Bridgeport, Connecticut.

Curriculum Surveys

Probably the first survey of dental hygiene education to be made by the Association was done in 1932 by the Committee on Dental Hygiene in an attempt to determine how many dental hygienists had graduated.

The following year the president recommended that a survey be made of all courses of dental hygiene in the various training schools and development of educational standards which might be endorsed by the ADHA. It was also suggested that a committee study dental practice acts and prepare a model law which might be used by the states, and that a survey be made of the numbers of dental hygienists in each area of practice. The committee gathered data about facts on curricular offerings, state department of education requirements, and dental practice act provisions and recommended that, since the survey was merely a beginning and the need for further investigation was urgent, the committee continue its assignment.

The curriculum survey made in 1935 reported that of fifty-four subjects taught, only five were common to all programs and that there was a diversity of opinions regarding the importance of various courses. For instance, general chemistry varied from 11 to 68 hours of lecture with 22 to 214 hours of laboratory work. Examinations were inconsistent as were requirements for employment in state departments of education. The committee recommended that credit from dental hygiene courses should be given toward a degree and that more uniform training would meet the needs not only of state educational programs but of all areas of dental hygiene practice.

A survey of "training" schools in 1939 showed that there were still discrepancies in course offerings. Two schools offered a four-year course leading to a degree, seven had two-year courses and one offered a one-year course with one more year optional. Some of the recommendations in the report were that all programs should be a minimum of two years, some subjects should be eliminated and others added, and one year of college work should be required prior to entrance into dental hygiene. It was not until 1944 that a committee was appointed to standardize the requirements for training for dental hygienists.

The committee next surveyed colleges and universities allowing credit for some dental hygiene courses toward a degree, asking what courses were required and what extension classes members should be encouraged to take. Graduates presented unique backgrounds in courses completed to the point that the committee found it practical to make overall recommendations and suggested that each person submit her credits to be evaluated by the desired school. Since few dental hygiene credits were transferable, the Association might try to gain recognition of these credits.

On the recommendation of the ADA Council on Dental Education, "Minimum Standards of the Education of the Dental Hygienist," providing for a minimum of two academic years of training at the level of a college discipline, were adopted by the ADA House of Delegates in 1947. While somewhat changed from the ADHA's original draft and recommendation, the goal had been achieved: minimum standards were adopted. All dental hygiene educational programs were a minimum of two years in 1950 and were working toward uniformity of curriculum and training.

A "Cost Analysis for the Establishment of a School, Curriculum or Department for Dental Hygiene Education" was completed in 1959. This information was distributed to the Board and was sent to the ADA Council on Dental Education and deans of schools having dental hygiene programs for their use and information.

Other curriculum surveys were made in 1951, 1958 and 1964 in preparation for or in response to conferences on dental hygiene education, each one showing progress toward the goals of the committee.

The Association's response to requests from administrators of both new and established programs for course outlines and curriculum outlines was development of "Curriculum Essentials." The Association has taken the view that there is no single best curriculum, and that the true measure of worth of an educational program or a teacher lies in the competence of graduating students. Curriculum essentials contain the minimum preparation for practice. The objectives are subject to revision after one year of use, and periodically thereafter, as professional trends alter curriculum needs.*

Funded by the Kellogg Foundation, two years in preparation, the first stage of the curriculum project was completed in late 1970 by a subcommittee of the Committee on Dental Hygiene Education with the assistance of Peter Pipe, Senior Associate of Pipe and Associates Consultants in Instructive Technology. Essential skills of the dental hygienist have been identified so that minimum preparation for practice can be outlined, establishing guidelines to standardize curriculums.

Since World War II, the dental hygienist trained by the military has helped to fill the need for preventive dental care in the services. This committee and the Committee on Legislation are now concerned with the development of mechanisms consistent with the current standards of quality dental hygiene education to provide for the transition from military to civilian practice. This would include evaluating existing knowledge and skills and providing supplemental education needed to qualify military trained personnel for licensure examination.

Division of Educational Services

The steadily increasing duties of the Committee on Dental Hygiene Education, and the prospect of more activities, made the Association aware of the need for growth and change in its structure. Volunteer members could not begin to administer activities in the area of dental hygiene education or provide the continuity and guidance required for this growing profession. Full-time staff was desperately needed to administer policies established by the Association. With the approval of the House of Delegates, the Committee on Dental Hygiene submitted a grant proposal to the W. K. Kellogg Foundation. Acceptance of the proposal allowed the establishment of the Division of Educational Services in 1967 under the supervision of a full-time director. The three-year funding provided for the

* Ad Hoc Committee on Curriculum, ADHA, 1970.

Association to assume an increasing share of costs, taking full financial responsibility at the end of the period.*

While the activities of the Division of Education, formerly the Division of Educational Services, are diversified, all of these activities are directed to two general goals:

1. The continued improvement and development of dental hygiene education programs. The need is recognized not only to produce dental hygienists capable of completing those procedures currently assigned to the dental hygienist but, also, to experiment with the dental hygiene curriculum in ways which will make it possible to prepare dental hygienists for additional responsibilities, and even cast some light on what some of those additional responsibilities will be. There is also a recognized need to develop programs of continuing education which will enable practicing dental hygienists to prepare themselves for additional duties and keep abreast of recent developments in the profession.

2. The other area to which the Division directs its attention is that of increased participation by the dental hygiene profession in establishing standards of quality and acceptability for dental hygiene. While the Council on Dental Education of the ADA will continue to be the accrediting body for dental hygiene education programs for the foreseeable future, excellent channels of liaison have been established with that organization.

Under the direction of the Division, "Admissions Requirements of Dental Hygiene Schools" was compiled and published by means of a grant from the American Fund for Dental Health, and a Clinical Dental Hygiene Teachers' Institute, also funded by the AFDH, was held in the summer of 1969. A Community Dental Health Teachers' Institute and a Radiology Teachers' Institute have been given and similar institutes are being planned. Through government contracts a Career Options Curriculum in Dentistry Study and a Dental Hygiene Education Assessment are nearing completion.

Conferences

The lack of information about the aims and objectives of dental hygiene education and about specific courses and types of training which could best provide the experience and education required made it impossible for formal inspections of existing dental hygiene schools to begin immediately after requirements for accreditation were approved. As a result, a "Conference on Teaching Programs for the Training of Dental Hygienists" was held in 1949. Representatives from the American Dental Hygienists' Association, American Association of Dental Examiners, American Association of Dental Schools, American Dental Association and schools eligible for inspection participated. A check list of about 350 skills and abilities that should be considered and evaluated was developed and was the first portion of a curriculum study on dental hygiene education.†

A second workshop was sponsored by the Council in 1951 to study in greater detail and to make recommendations about the aims and objectives of dental hygiene education, the needs of curriculum and the development

* Committee Reports, ADHA, 1966-1967.
† Workshop on Dental Education and Licensure. Proceedings, October 1964.

of certain minimum standards. Accreditation procedures were formulated from statements developed on each dental hygiene course, clinical teaching, basic science teaching, admission requirements, library, physical facilities, faculty and finances.*

A third conference, in 1955, devoted to studying course content of basic science courses, also discussed and approved the concept of aptitude and achievement testing to study and evaluate the effectiveness of teaching programs and to improve admissions procedures. It was believed an achievement testing program would have potential value to licensing boards and that it might become the basis for National Board examinations in dental hygiene.*

A fourth conference on dental hygiene education in 1961, although originally planned to review results of the achievement testing program, was restructured to discuss the newly authorized establishment of the National Board examination. The potential of the achievement test had been proven and it did become the basis for the National Board examination in dental hygiene.*

The Council on Dental Education, American Association of Dental Schools and American Dental Hygienists' Association, believing that it was time for a reevaluation of responsibilities and functions of the dental hygienist, sponsored the 1964 Conference on Dental Hygiene Education and Licensure. Each dental and dental hygiene education program, each state board of dental examiners, each constituent dental and dental hygiene society, the United States Public Health Service and the W. K. Kellogg Foundation were invited to send a representative. Participants reexamined the present and considered potential duties and responsibilities of the dental hygienist, evaluated the adequacy of present requirements for education and proposed revisions indicated in licensure regulations for dental hygienists.*

This was followed by a Conference for Dental Hygiene Educators sponsored by the ADHA in 1965. Outlined goals were to identify present and potential responsibilities dental hygiene students must learn to assume in terms of clinical, educational and community services; definition of the degree of competency dental hygiene students must learn to assume in order to be graduated; establishment of better mechanisms for better communications between administrators and professional colleagues.†

The increased demand for dental auxiliary services and potential expansion of duties created the need for the 1967 workshop, again sponsored by the ADHA, to redefine standards and objectives of two-year certificate, baccalaureate and graduate programs in dental hygiene. Policy statements were subsequently adopted by the House of Delegates and have been updated to meet changing needs of dental hygiene education.‡

* Ibid.
† Conference for Dental Hygiene Educators. Proceedings, April 1965.
‡ Workshop in Undergraduate and Graduate Programs in Dental Hygiene. Proceedings, July 1967.

On a more limited attendance basis the Association has held indoctrination conferences for its regional consultants to dental hygiene programs and conducted a clinical teachers' institute.

Accreditation

In 1947 the ADHA Committee on Education for Dental Hygienists, composed of representatives from schools of dental hygiene, Frances Stoll, chairman, drafted and submitted minimum standards for the education of the dental hygienist to the ADA Council on Dental Education. At the annual session a panel of dentists discussed accreditation, requirements, establishment of a school and standardization of laws required for licensure and education. The discussion emphasized the need for a study of laws, curriculum, practice and increased course length to two years.

ADHA representatives met with the ADA Council on Dental Education prior to accreditation visits to help establish procedures. These meetings were sponsored by the American Dental Association, the American Association of Dental Schools and the American Dental Hygienists' Association. A definition of the functions of the dental hygienist was adopted as a basis for determining curriculum requirements. Other meetings considered admissions, plant, equipment, faculty, organization and administration, library, financial support, clinical and basic science teaching, and research. The data were gathered from directors of schools in order that criteria would have sound bases.

After revision by the ADA Council on Dental Education these criteria were submitted to and approved by the ADA House of Delegates. The first accreditation visits were made in 1952 by a committee composed of two representatives from the Council, one representative from the ADHA, and one representative from the state board of dental examiners of the appropriate jurisdictions.

Recruitment of qualified applicants has long been an Association concern. The first admission requirements stipulated "one year past the 8th grade," which was changed through the efforts of the Association to "high school graduate." In an attempt to recruit qualified applicants, and at the suggestion of the ADA, aptitude testing as a screening process was studied in 1955. Achievement tests were a logical follow-up to the aptitude test and were used as pilot studies for National Board Examinations in dental hygiene.

The Committee on Dental Hygiene Education considered admissions testing programs and when the scope of this activity became apparent, a sub-committee was formed for this one purpose. The Psychological Corporation, which eventually operated the program, worked with Mrs. Frances Dolan, chairman, and members of the new sub-committee, organizing aptitude and achievement test procedures. Shailer Peterson and Mrs. Grace Parkin, Council on Dental Education staff members, also assisted the sub-committee. Funds for a three-year pilot program were obtained from the Kellogg Foundation.

A list of dental hygienists recommended by the ADHA Committee on Dental Hygiene Education and approved by the Board is submitted each year to the ADA Council on Dental Education for selection to assist in accreditation procedures. The many new programs to be evaluated in addition to the periodic evaluation of established programs have increased the number of ADHA members who participate in this activity.

National Board Examinations

National Board Dental Hygiene Examinations were inaugurated in 1962. They are conducted by the Council of National Board Dental Examiners of the American Dental Association and are a joint project of the American Dental Association, American Association of Dental Examiners, American Association of Dental Schools and American Dental Hygienists' Association. A Council sub-committee composed of three members of the Council and four dental hygiene consultants recommends rules and regulations for administration of the examination. These examinations are conducted as a service to the dental and dental hygiene professions and ultimately to help maintain a high standard of dental care for the public.

Many dental hygienists have been lost to the health manpower force through marriage or moving to states where licenses were not held. In the belief that this situation could be alleviated if there were a mechanism whereby dental hygienists could become licensed without unreasonable study and reexamination, a liaison committee was appointed in 1958 to work with the ADA Council of National Board of Dental Examiners and the American Association of Dental Examiners. Their task was to develop an examination for dental hygienists that would be accepted by all examining bodies. The first examination was administered in 1962 and all states except Delaware, New Jersey and the Territory of Puerto Rico accepted the National Board Examination in Dental Hygiene by 1970.

Four dental hygienists, two private practitioners and two dental hygiene educators, were appointed to serve on the ADA National Board Committee on a rotating basis. Margaret Ryan and Lucille Klein, representing private practice, and Louise Hord and Rebekah Fisk representing dental hygiene education were the first appointees. Miss Ryan, by then first vice president of the ADHA, was appointed as chairman of the Dental Hygiene Committee, Council of National Board of Dental Examiners in 1965.

The National Board Examination in Dental Hygiene was a multiple-choice examination over twelve subject areas, divided into four sections:

1. General Anatomy, Dental Anatomy, Physiology
2. Histology, Pathology, Roentgenology
3. Chemistry, Nutrition, Microbiology
4. Pharmacology, Dental Materials, Preventive Aspects of Dentistry

Responding to changing needs of the profession the National Board Examination became a comprehensive examination in 1973. It contains 400 items and is administered during a six-hour period in a single day and draws on knowledge directly related to clinical functions performed by dental hygienists. Review will be made by state licensing boards, dental hygiene schools and the full Council.*

The number of student candidates has more than doubled since the first year while the number of graduate candidates has decreased sharply. The 1970 examination produced the highest reliability coefficient of any examination since 1962.

Continuing Education

Continuing education, briefly defined, is education by formal courses or other Association-approved means after the basic dental hygiene education has been completed. It is accepted today as one means of ensuring high quality and continued competence of the dental hygienist. Many continuing education courses are presented in all areas of the United States, but, while they are well attended, they do not reach all dental hygienists. The 1969 House of Delegates recommended that the Committee on Dental Hygiene Education direct its attention to the standards and mechanisms for continuing education as it pertains to licensure renewal. This it is doing through an Ad Hoc Committee. Some states have already incorporated this concept into their laws; others are considering this action. A few state Associations include similar requirements in qualification for membership.

Continuing education, a primary concern today, was first mentioned in the *Journal* of May, 1927. The University of Buffalo for the second year offered a six-week postgraduate course "by the advice and through the co-operation of the New York State Department of Education." Courses for which dental hygienists could register were: Education (Principles of Teaching); Child Psychology; Public Speaking; Applied Oral Hygiene (Field Problems); Nutrition; and, according to the *Journal:* "other related courses in education are available and can be substituted for any already taken."

Trends in Dental Hygiene

The 1960's have seen the beginning of dramatic changes in all health professions. As spokesman for dental hygiene the Association must know the desires of its membership and be able to relay these facts to appropriate agencies. Among dental hygienists there are differing viewpoints and interests because of the various fields of practice. The Association must have sensitivity, for its response to these differences is essential. Much of the expression of this sensitivity depends on the elected officers and the executive director.

* Committee Reports, ADHA, 1923-1974.

A 1939 survey of members showed that less than 10 per cent of responding dental hygienists had duties limited to prophylaxis, 90 per cent were responsible for secretarial work, 70 per cent exposed radiographs, 65 per cent were required to do chairside assisting and laboratory procedures and 12 per cent assisted in administration of nitrous oxide, some responsible for the whole procedure. Forty per cent were taking further educational courses, some to earn degrees.

A later survey, in 1948, showed that the majority of dental hygienists (56 per cent) were in private practice and the duties of only 10 per cent of them were limited to the dental prophylaxis. Other duties assigned included secretarial work, radiography, chairside assisting, reception, bookkeeping and laboratory procedures. School dental clinics employed approximately 26 per cent of the responding dental hygienists, and the remainder were divided among state and federal civil service, teaching, industrial clinics, hospitals, institutional clinics, armed services and part-time practice. Ninety per cent of the respondents believed that their training was inadequate, and 40 per cent were taking additional courses to remedy this defect. Salaries were highest in industrial clinics, lowest in school clinics.

A 1962 survey concerning professional trends was undertaken to determine (1) what responsibilities dental hygienists were currently undertaking, and (2) their attitudes toward undertaking certain other responsibilities under supervision of a dentist after proper training and providing these new responsibilities were made legal by dental practice acts. The questionnaire also aroused interest in the fact that expanded services were being discussed and considered.

Eighty per cent of those responding were in private practice; other areas included pedodontic practice, periodontal practice, government, departments of education, hospitals and dental hygiene education. Seventy-two per cent attended two-year dental hygiene programs; the remainder had three, four or more years of college education. Returned questionnaires showed that the majority of dental hygienists were interested in performing expanded functions in preventive and educative procedures but not in restorative procedures.

A Special Task Force Committee of the ADHA, representing dental hygiene education, private practice and community dental health areas, was appointed in 1966 to study social, political and economic trends affecting dental and dental hygiene practice, as well as dental hygiene manpower and its relationship to members of the dental health team.

Dental hygienists are aware of changing trends in the delivery of health care services. The Liaison Committee with the American Association of Dental Examiners has brought the inconsistencies between dental hygiene practice and dental hygiene legislation to the attention of the states. The AADE has encouraged changes in dental practice acts to enable rather than inhibit dental hygiene practice so that rules and regulations of individual state boards of dentistry will guide the delegation of duties by the dentist to his auxiliary personnel.

As early as 1948 the ADHA House of Delegates adopted a policy which stated that until the American Dental Association indicates its desire that dental hygienists assume additional duties, the ADHA opposes any increase in the field of practice but, that when such duties are delegated, dental hygienists are the logical choice of auxiliary personnel. In the early 1960's the ADA adopted a policy that encouraged the establishment in accredited dental schools of experimental programs to study expansion of duties of auxiliary personnel. The need for the Association to develop strong, reasonable policies on current issues of expansion of duties, licensure and continuing education is recognized. If something must be opposed, reasonable alternatives must be suggested. A continuing study of objectives, new roles to be assumed and problems of the future has been undertaken. Under the direction of the Committee on Dental Hygiene Education a broad policy statement was presented to and approved by the 1968 House of Delegates. In summary the statement recognized that there was an increased need for preventive and restorative dental services for the public which could be met in part by more effective utilization of the dental hygienist; that the dental hygienist's services primarily should be preventive; that if predicated on educational preparation, state licensure could assure dentistry and the public of quality services; that licensure renewal should be based on preparation for these extended duties. A 1970 revision acknowledged that the practice of dental hygiene could be extended into restorative areas: "the American Dental Hygienists' Association, recognizing the continued need to meet increasing demands for dental services, reaffirms its support of the delegation of additional duties, including both preventive and restorative, to dental hygienists and its belief that such delegation of duties be based on competence resulting from specific education."

The House of Delegates approved a request to the ADA for formation of a joint committee of dental and dental auxiliary groups to explore the potential expansion of auxiliaries' duties. In 1970 the Interagency Task Force Committee, whose members represented the ADA Council on Dental Education, The American Dental Hygienists' Association, American Dental Assistants Association, American Association of Dental Examiners and American Association of Dental Schools, met and drafted recommendations which were submitted to the Council on Dental Education.

The American Dental Hygienists' Association has maintained acceptance and liaison and established working relationships with the American Dental Association and other allied health groups. In addition to representation on the National Board Dental Hygiene Examinations, the ADHA formally participates in accreditation of schools of dental hygiene and provides educational consultants for new programs of dental hygiene, and Board members serve on liaison committees with allied groups.

Top priority currently is being given to an in-depth study of the present and future needs of dental hygiene education, undergraduate, graduate and continuing education opportunities; legislation affecting the profession of dental hygiene; and the extension of duties of auxiliary personnel. Project Alliance, a study made in 1971, reassessed the goals of the Association and identified areas of common interest in which this Association could work in advantageous cooperation with related oral health auxiliary organizations. Formal and informal participation in all these areas increases each year and there is every reason to believe that these trends will continue.

Through concern for the dental health of the public, service to dentistry and commitment to its membership, the American Dental Hygienists' Association is fulfilling its destiny as the instrument to make dental hygiene "a great and continuously progressive profession."

References

History of the Connecticut Dental Hygienists' Association. JADHA, 5:26, 1931.

Ohio State Dental Hygienists' Association: History and progress of dental hygiene in the United States. JADHA, 1:3-9, 1927.

Junck, Anita, and Barney, Elizabeth: A glance backward. Northern California State Dental Hygienists' Association, 1964.

Minutes of the ADHA, 1923-1974.

Myers, Sharon E.: WHO and dental auxiliaries around the world. JADHA, 4:3, 1970.

Operations and Procedures Manual, ADHA, 1970.

Bylaws, ADHA, 1970.

McCain, Diane: Objectives and responsibilities of the Washington office. ADHA, 1971.

Ad-Hoc Committee on Curriculum, ADHA, 1970.

Committee Reports, ADHA, 1923-1974.

Workshop on Dental Hygiene Education and Licensure, Proceedings, October 1964.

Conference for Dental Hygiene Educators, Proceedings, April 1965.

Workshop on Undergraduate and Graduate Programs in Dental Hygiene, Proceedings, July 1967.

Chapter 7

Challenges of Contemporary Ethics

Responsibility to Everyday Ethical Challenges

"Crisis" is from the Greek *krinen,* to judge, and then *krisis,* the decisive moment. The Chinese ideogram for "crisis" is composed of the characters representing "danger" and "opportunity." A crisis, in any language, then, can be the turning point for progress or decadence. As an example, dealing with student unrest presents the danger of aggravating physical violence and destruction of property, but it also offers the challenge of finding a peaceful, constructive solution.

Man has not been able to synchronize his social consciousness with the rapid accumulation and application of scientific knowledge which has accelerated the tempo of all life. As a result, new value conflicts have been created and values are rightfully being examined and questioned.

Many of the world's present difficulties and problems can be attributed to outdated institutions and thinking. In part, this unwillingness to alter attitudes can be charged to vested interests which do not encourage change beneficial to the general public if such change involves a lessening of a monetary return. Another factor contributing to the apparent reluctance to modernize attitudes is the general complacency of the "Great American Public." There are too many people who are blindly satisfied with human affairs as they are and only when their personal security is threatened, and then often with great protest, are they motivated to even consider change. Those who care and are concerned must have courage and security within themselves so that they can support measures to overcome these obstacles.

Defining the challenges of ethics encountered in everyday living by labeling them as "issues" or "problems" indicates that they have not yet been resolved by responsible actions. At least, dispositions of the problems have not been accepted by the majority of people and have not yet had time to affect behavior and mores in general. The good and the evil embodied in ethical challenges are intrinsically different and are based on more than individual preferences. If good and evil were merely personal preferences there would be no need to try to persuade someone to change his belief and accept another, for there is no argument against the fact that tastes differ.

It must be realized that all value judgments reflect personal bias, for judgments are based on the individual's frame of reference which includes present knowledge, previous experiences and the ability to reason logically. It must also be noted that dissent can be valid and is not necessarily evidence of malice or stupidity. Indeed, if there is no dissent then, in effect, we would say that all people, all relationships, all institutions, all systems, all governments, all business, all professions and all other concerns are as good as they can be. Obviously this is not so, for there is much room for improvement in present world relationships and no one would want to preclude discoveries or advances in knowledge and their applications to human affairs. Informed, peaceful dissent is a healthy state and should be encouraged at all levels of society.

Those people who are committed to a cause or ideal are likely to have very definite opinions for they have studied the problem and reached a considered conclusion; however, strong loyalties do not necessarily blind them to the possible alternatives. Bigots, who are unwilling to listen to another viewpoint, and blind partisans, who follow a cause without tempered thought, represent the extremes of passions and prejudices to which some people subscribe.

Persuasion is the tool most often used to bring about changes in ethical attitudes. Facts, as persuaders, can sometimes be used to advantage by citing statistics compiled before and after some action has been taken. However, accumulated figures and obscured facts are not applicable to all issues for some of them go deeper and involve standards of value. Standards, rightly applied, then become crucial in the resolution of issues.

Flower-children of the 1960's rejected middle-class values of work and ambition which bring material possessions and status, and substituted a free-loading existence and escape from reality in drugs. Their differences with the rest of the world were basically over standards and ideals, matters which are value judgments.

Concerned people must be able to consider alternatives to such pseudo solutions. They must be willing to stand back from the situation and with clear minds reevaluate the issue from viewpoints not previously considered. Then, and only then, can there be an intelligent reaffirmation of value standards or, if necessary, a revision of these standards so they will conform to the new criteria. Individuals submissive to the group would not dare to make such a challenge, so the close and impersonal examination of value judgments is clearly an exercise of free will.

Many commitments in today's complex world compete for attention and there are constant demands on the dental hygienist's time and energy. Organizations dedicated to solving problems facing dentistry, society, city, state and federal government involve all of the people to some degree and frustrate them at times because they are not able to contribute and accomplish as much as desired. There are many ways by which the dental hygienist may achieve personal fulfillment. Some individuals find that only one area of involvement will satisfy them; others need more than one source for gratification. A multifaceted approach is not only desirable but perhaps indispensable in our modern societal structure. The union of diverse interests to accomplish seemingly insurmountable challenges is needed today more than ever before.

The challenges presented in the following pages of this chapter are far from a complete list of all ethical questions of the contemporary world; they are merely representative. Nor are they discussed at any length, or in depth, for each issue could be a volume in itself. Further, the challenges made are timely as written, but timely material rapidly becomes outdated. Although an attempt has been made to present viewpoints, no conclusions are drawn; each individual must make his own informed decisions. While some will have very definite opinions on these and other issues, their opinions are often one-sided because few people have had, or used, the opportunity to study all the ramifications of ethical challenges. These discussions are primarily intended as stimuli to promote further examination and consideration.

Challenge: Internal Security

How far should the federal government go in establishing and maintaining national security, in preventing civil revolution, in protecting the people from disruptive forces? What are the boundaries between individual rights and governmental rights? How much personal liberty must be given up in order to secure protection of other rights?

In past years the term "civil strife" brought to the mind of the United States citizen internal order within the confines of the United States or one of its segments, but, today, civil strife is rampant on a worldwide basis and no person, group or government is exempt from involvement in some manner. Today's world demands that a workable way of ordering social relationships encompassing the whole world population be found.

Is revolution ever morally justified? If it is, then under what conditions? After years of "taxation without representation," but not without careful consideration punctuated by impassioned pleas for and cautionary speeches against, the Declaration of Independence was written, signed and adopted by representatives of the colonies. If it were not for this revolution fomented by colonial patriots, and supported by outside governments, the United States of America would not have become an independent entity in 1776. Right or wrong, this revolution has been immortalized, with pride, in American history and literature. And many of today's citizens, if they had been alive and living in France, might have been members of the crowd which stormed the Bastille on July 14, 1789.

The Revolutionary War provides early examples of security measures and individual moral decisions made during time of war. In 1776 the British accused Nathan Hale of being a spy and promptly executed him. His words, made famous in history, "I only regret that I have but one life to give for my country," give insight into the firm convictions about independence, liberty and patriotism that he and many early colonists had. Benedict Arnold, on the other hand, let his personal pique take precedence over loyalty to his country. Annoyed by a reprimand from General Washington, he decided deliberately to turn traitor and give West Point to the British. He escaped and fought with the British army, but lost his United States citizenship.

The specter of communism was one of the first modern-day disruptive influences of federal internal security. Measures taken to guard this security included requiring signed loyalty oaths from certain classes of employees. Some signed willingly for they were loyal to their country and were, in addition, law abiding. Party communists probably signed without compunction over the fact that they were being dishonest in doing so. But a third group objected to signing loyalty oaths on the grounds that this was in conflict with the personal liberties and rights guaranteed by the Constitution.

Another unresolved issue of current interest also has to do with laws. Are people obliged to obey a law which they are convinced is morally wrong? Is the law of the land always supreme? Should citizens be law abiding and violate their consciences, or should they follow the dictates of conscience and personal mores and violate the law, when in either case they are contradicting some part of their beliefs? To have respect for a law, one must have respect for what the law does. Is there always a dominant conviction or can people have contradictory beliefs? When Socrates was ordered by the court to stop teaching philosophy, his belief in the rightness of his action not only kept him teaching but also kept him from running away from the consequences of his decision and ultimately led to his death.

Because man lives in a free society he may make his own judgment about the competence of any duly constituted authority, whether this authority is vested in a person or a law, and he may express his opinion freely. Many courses of action may be sanctioned by morality but not by law. However, in an orderly society man cannot expect the protection of the law when he decides that he cannot cooperate with a particular law. He may seek protection through the law, but it is not his as a matter of right.

There are two ways by which the individual can protest what he feels is an unjust law—he can passively wait for a change to be effected by law makers, or he may protest the law, either peacefully or violently, alone or collectively.

Henry Thoreau, an early American example of protest against what he believed to be an inappropriate law, refused to pay taxes. His reasoning was that the government which received that tax money was spending it to finance the war with Mexico, a war which Thoreau felt was unjust; in addition, the government was tolerating slavery, a condition which was abhorrent to him. In one of his writings on the subject he posed the rhetorical question that, if man has been given an individual conscience, then why must this conscience be resigned to legislators? Mahatma Gandhi studied Thoreau's writings and philosophy and adapted parts of them to augment his own philosophy, by which he influenced the populace of India to use passive resistance as a tool.

In the judicial system of the United States the constitutionality of a law cannot be determined until it is challenged and brought to court for a decision, but frequently it cannot be brought to court until it is violated. Often some individual citizen, or a group, will make a technical violation merely for the sake of creating a test case. During recent years blacks have resorted to this device to bring attention to the inequalities of their treatment despite new laws affecting them favorably. Dentists employing dental hygienists have also used technical violation as a device to force legislators to make legal provision for the practice of dental hygiene.

Challenge: Minority Groups

Were the basic freedom and equality guaranteed in the Constitution of the United States meant for everybody? Apparently not all the founding fathers thought so. Although the Civil War was an attempt to settle the dispute between those who were eager to abolish slavery and those who wanted to retain the institution, in actuality it aided in rejecting the premise of the inherent inferiority of the black race in America. Slavery was a social problem for slaves and an ethical problem for slave holders. Neither problem was solved by legislation. Today, through a more developed social consciousness, the precept of slavery, that one man can "own" another, has been rejected. But has there been an honest attempt made to find acceptable solutions for the social problems connected with wholehearted acceptance of the black population? Isn't western civilization still thinking in conditioned dichotomies, believing that dark-skinned and other minority groups, per se, are inferior, therefore they (the white-skinned group) must be superior? It is an obvious conclusion to many of the majority group. But this conclusion is one of fallacy, not fact.

Discrimination has shown itself in many ways. There have been the flaunted discriminations of levying poll taxes and requiring proof of literacy for voting procedures, restrictions which forced people of minority groups to live in ghettos or other undesirable areas, and hiring based on race, sex or creed rather than on ability. Discrimination can be more subtle but just as effective when a right, enforced for one group, forces another group to relinquish some right. Sometimes the law, although well meaning, has been a hindrance rather than a help to minority groups. As an example, the racism of the South has been greatly dependent on the law which forced all persons, regardless of their thoughts or feelings to practice racial segregation.

The black man has become a cause célèbre because he has maximized his complaints and demands more vocally than other minority groups who have also been repressed or neglected. It is true that the United States offered more opportunity than many other lands for the foreign-born family to raise its standard of living, and thus encouraged migration to this country. But has there really been equal opportunity given to all these people? First-generation American born children of these families accepted their parents' way of living because of ancestral influences. Later generations, encouraged by changing attitudes and realizing their deprivations, are raising their voices in an attempt to secure equal rights for themselves. Quality education, better housing and job opportunities are prime targets for improvement.

Law and education are the bases of freedom and equal opportunity, and undisciplined violence or unreasonable demands made by minority groups will not help them to attain their stated goal of equality. Laws must be just, based on precepts which ignore race, creed or sex, and such laws must be administered impartially. Education must be able to persuade people to acknowledge the universality of human dignity of all individuals and to encourage a personal sense of worth and responsibility.

Expectations of improvement have been raised and encouraged, but not enough action has been taken. It is easy to talk about and bemoan inequalities, easy to acknowledge relevant facts as an indictment of a wrong system. It is also easy to lose interest in taking corrective measures. Action is difficult for it takes true moral conviction and dedication to continue against the odds of apathy, time, bigotry and even punishment. Equality in all respects can never be ensured, because natural capacities vary, but the basic freedoms to choose friends, to control personal and family life, to participate competitively in an economic system and in a social system of free association, can be ensured—as can the equality of voting, administration of justice and access to public services. If the Constitution was really meant to "secure the blessings of liberty," and if the individual conscience is activated, then everyone, regardless of race, creed or sex, should be free to be different in his ambitions and abilities.

Challenge: Right of Privacy

With the increasing role of government at all levels in financial support of health needs it becomes incumbent on those government agencies to accept the responsibility of protecting the right of privacy of each and every person. The confidentiality of health information needs to be maintained. Virtually every common "release of medical information" form today gives *carte blanche* to the doctor, hospital, laboratory and even the pharmacist to relate what they know about the patient. The patient is sole owner of these details, and the doctor or hospital merely custodians, and he should have the right to know and give approval of any medical information which is shared. Most people have no idea of what is being said about them, or to whom, or even if the data are accurate. Third party agencies seem to find ways of securing what should be confidential information.

There should be guidelines agreed upon which would establish a statute of limitations on certain types of information and delineate areas relating to subpoenas, disclosure of credit information, psychiatric records and the rights of patients to have access to their own records. These guidelines should not restrict or interfere with the free exchange of medical information between medical agents or agencies.

Questions to be resolved include who is to have access to medical records; how to use them and perhaps more important, how not to use them.

Challenge: The Conscientious Objector

Since all people are in one way or another personally affected by wars, another debatable issue is the stand of the conscientious objector. In 1917 members of the religious groups of Friends, Mennonites and Brethren were exempted from bearing arms in war, although they served in non-combatant capacities and not all members took advantage of the provision. The legal decision was based on the reasoning that all war was in violation of the religious training of these sects. The Universal Military Training Act was passed in 1948 to allow anyone with deep convictions of the wrongness of war to be exempt from active combat service. In an attempt to clarify this somewhat ambiguous statement, the Supreme Court in 1965 said that Congress did not mean to require a belief in God for exemption, although it did not specify exactly what other grounds were acceptable.

The religious conscientious objector is opposed to all killing; the pacifist takes sides in a conflict but affirms the futility of war; the neutralist believes that the good and evil of the war at hand are too evenly balanced for him to be able to take sides. The selective conscientious objector might object to all wars or just to a particular war, for the tactics being used or for the economic or political factors involved.

Some conscientious objectors, although not bearing arms, have served in dangerous areas on battlefields or have participated in medical research, but others have left the United States, apparently willing to renounce loyalty to their country, preferring to give up their citizenship rather than serve in a non-combatant capacity or to submit to a jail sentence for evasion of duty. What is the highest duty: duty to one's own ethical beliefs or duty to laws of the land?

During the war in Vietnam objecting youths, decrying war, believed that they were justified in preventing employee recruitment by manufacturers of war supplies or in interfering with activities of military training programs. Equal rights giving individuals the freedom of choice are thus utterly ignored.

The President in 1974 offered amnesty to those who had fled to other countries. Is this fair to those who served honorably, many of whom gave their lives, or those who paid penalties in other ways?

Can any or all of these attitudes be justified morally or legally?

Challenge: Crime and Punishment

Citizens vested with the right to own property individually attempt to protect themselves from thieves and from bodily assault. Police departments have been created and the responsibility for this protection has been delegated to them. The question, then, is to what extent should law enforcement agencies perform necessary acts involved with this duty? How many and which individual rights should citizens be willing to give up in order to secure protection for person and property?

No society can exist without the use of coercion, but the least amount possible should be used. Not all citizens can be trusted to obey laws or act ethically, but through fear of penalties (a peaceful coercion) they comply. Police, in addition to enforcing laws, are a peaceful threat to complacent individuals who would not otherwise follow any reforms or pay taxes.

A penal system is provided for use when other measures fail to halt law breaking. In addition to protecting the citizen from harm, this system was meant to deter the individual from committing a first offense and to reform or correct an offender, but it also punishes justly or unjustly. Statistics show that punishment has not been very effective as a deterrent or as a reform mechanism. One of the most difficult problems of ethics is defining the difference between blame and blamelessness: was the act committed with free will or was it conduct over which there was no control? While our criminal reform system appears to be in transition, headed for better understanding of alternatives and necessities, society seems to believe in punishment for its own sake. Is it being childishly vindictive to subscribe to the theory that the way to deal with criminals is to punish them, or is this really the only way to correct them?

Contrary to opinion, punishment is not a universal solvent, for some people are unable to learn and reactions differ. Prisons are known as the best schools for learning the trade of crime, and punishment may make the person more careful to avoid discovery of his next crime rather than to live within the law. Psychologists state that it is possible to predict with a high percentage of accuracy which offenders will repeat their crimes and which will not. With this in mind, would it be better to accept the lifetime care of constant offenders than to release them and risk the possibility of injury or death of innocent persons? Capital punishment will continue to be a controversial, ethical topic of discussion. In spite of all the arguments for and against the death penalty, it might be well to consider giving the accused person a choice so that he may preserve his personal dignity in his own way.

Surveys show that the public believes the current correctional system is inadequate but people are not eager for change if it means more money would be spent. Also, the public today is less inclined toward punishment and tends to look to rehabilitation—but is not tolerant toward the returned offender.

Many people have had problems and either have had help in solving them or were strong enough to survive in a socially acceptable manner. Others have not been able to manage by themselves. These are the people who need special help to live up to society's expectations for citizenship. We must cope with today's criminal, but in the future perhaps enlightened citizens should look more seriously to the "why" of antisocial behavior instead of concentrating on the crime and its punishment. If, as Karl Menninger says, people are failures first, criminals later, how much better to concentrate on means of avoiding failures.

New interpretations of the law seem to require a lesser or no penalty assessed against the criminal. The private citizen therefore has less protection and less recourse. Another question being reviewed is equal application of the law. Are the wealthy and the government official to be exempt from penalties levied on the ordinary citizen for the commission of the same crime?

Challenge: Ethics of the Business Community

The ethics of the business community are related to two distinct yet interdependent issues: social obligation and honesty. In simple terms, honesty is not cheating, lying or stealing. Businesses cannot be social service agencies, but they can contribute meaningfully to this movement. While honesty and social obligation would not seem to be perplexing questions, close examination proves they are. At least close adherence to precepts is a shadowy area of business ethics.

Social responsibility is an undefined area of the corporate image. There are not likely to be standards of responsibility until there are clearly defined obligations in such areas as: how much responsibility should business accept for its workers; should a plant be allowed to dispose of waste products in a manner which upsets the ecology of the area, or should it accept added expense in other means of disposal; should manufacturers continue to market products such as insecticides and laundry detergents which also upset some areas of ecology, or do the beneficial effects of these products offset this aspect; should corporations aid churches and institutions of higher learning?

Every business must set up priorities, both physical and financial, and choose between frivolous expenditure and fundamental needs. But whose interests come first—private interests of management, or public interests of stockholders, employees and consumers? Majority rule, a precept accepted by Americans, can be a fallacy, for a minority pressure group is too often "the power behind the throne" in making such decisions. Too many individuals are more eager to have their Cadillacs and color television sets than they are willing to give up any bit of profit in exchange for such vital things as better schools and roads.

It is the obvious aim of a corporation to produce maximum profits for its stockholders but this must not be at the expense of its employees if it expects to survive. Any business endeavor is obligated to the community for its very existence, for it is the community which supplies the environment as well as the employees who are the labor force. This creates a responsibility to contribute to the welfare of the community through financial aid to higher education, to scientific, social or economic research and to charitable projects as well as other forms of support to these agencies. Personal involvement, not just gifts of money, is necessary to achieve the most productive relations between business and the community. John W. Gardner, as president of a foundation, required his staff to take one day a week, not nights or week ends, to devote themselves to something they were interested in outside the office. He claimed as a result the work of the organization improved as did the quality of his staff and the relationships with the community.

It has never been the American way to have as leader just one powerful person or clique; instead, our society thrives best on a variety of leadership. Traditionally Americans are against a welfare state—not against welfare for those who need help, but against a centralization of power. In addition, the welfare state leaves little room for personal idealism and, although it satisfies the anxieties of the middle-aged, it stifles the creativeness of the young. Business and government provide checks and balances for each other when some functions are assumed by each. Government, business, labor and agriculture rightly have differences of opinion and none becomes or remains dominant for long.

The law of the jungle often prevails in the business community and in the beginning, but perhaps only in theory, the business man was thought to be controlled by the market; it was felt that neither government nor moral leaders were needed to restrain him in his policies and his dealing with employees and the public. The demands and interests of labor and consumer were considered because business had to live with both of them. Today's market, dominated by corporate giants, is restrained to some degree by government-imposed standards of conduct through antitrust and labor laws and labor union contracts.

The human frailty of business executives should be no justification for a lowering of morals in any form, yet we see dishonesty in business in many ways. Expediency is often set above principle; there is lack of truth in advertising; advantage is taken of minority groups because of their lack of understanding of language and law; the expense account is padded, a conflict of interest is resolved for political or financial gain. Codes of ethics for many groups have been written or proposed but most of these codes are phrased in rather nebulous language and no enforcement techniques are available. Unless the individuals involved are subject to their own good consciences, or are under pressures of public opinion, the average individual will cheat.

Should everyone be allowed to strike, or is this privilege reserved for a chosen few? If not everyone can utilize this leverage mechanism to obtain desired benefits are equal rights violated? Are health professionals and public utilities workers exempt from this activity? What determines who can and who cannot strike? In past years those who offer service which affects the health of the public did not withdraw those services. Today's morality leans toward the fact that those workers, as much as anyone else, are entitled to fair remuneration and if arbitration with employers does not produce satisfactory results, withdrawal of service is acceptable. But who determines "satisfactory?" Does this violate the moral obligation of the health professional? Does self come first? Unions are bargaining agents for groups. They are not concerned with professional morals but the human rights of those they represent.

Challenge: Television

Is television's effect on culture good or bad? What are the moral responsibilities of the networks? When a television program is good there is nothing better. News reports, travelogues, educational and really entertaining programs can be of great value to the public. However, seventeen per cent of air time is devoted to commercial announcements, most of them not aimed at the public taste. While polls seem to give a boost to ratings of poor programs, these figures represent only those people who are watching at the moment of tabulation. There is nothing said about how many sets have been turned off or tuned in to another channel, so there are no figures to contradict the survey.

It has been estimated that during pre-kindergarten years the hours spent in watching television are greater than the hours spent in the first six years of school. And, further, a child spends as much time watching the television screen as he spends in school. This would indicate that the networks might be expected to have some moral obligation to upgrade the quality of programming to teach the child the alphabet as well as cereal names. They can easily add to the culture and give the viewer a wider selection of material.

Programs which provide relaxation, programs which meet the needs, not the whims, of the vocal public would be a significant public service. International television programs present an image to people of other countries, and few of these people really know Americans. What are they learning about the average citizen of the United States? Are they receiving an image that makes Americans proud or is it an embarrassingly inaccurate, distorted image? Television should be challenged to real leadership.

In spite of shortcomings, television is the medium which offers all people the opportunity to be eyewitnesses to historic events. Sharing the moon exploration at the instant of happening was one of the greatest examples of communication the world has ever experienced. The total presence of sight and sound and emotion, producing a feeling of kinship with all mankind, was made possible by a gigantic cooperative effort which included television.

Challenge: Advertising

Advertising is more than putting a company, product name or trademark before the public. It is persuasion in both open and subliminal ways. It can be a rational argument or pure propaganda; it is indispensable to business, but not always necessarily desirable to the public interest. The advertising copy writer studies human weaknesses, desires and fears in order to take advantage of public ignorance and to exploit public credulity. Is today's cynicism, which undoubtedly would have shocked earlier generations, to be continued or should advertising be pressured into honesty?

Vance Packard's *The Hidden Persuaders* amazes more readers than it horrifies because most people are resigned to advertising methods rather than becoming indignant about them. As examples, cosmetics commonly contain lanolin, which is good, and also cheap, but the manufacturers of beauty preparations, wrote one of their number, are selling "hope" not lanolin, and therefore receive a high price for their products. Much toothpaste is sold not as a cleansing agent for the teeth but as a guarantee against being repulsive through "bad breath" or "dingy teeth," or as a promise of instant sex-appeal. Automobiles reputedly give prestige and citrus products build vitality. A "grain" of truth is included, to be sure, but only an infinitesimal part of the whole.

Advertising knows that if a statement is made often enough people believe it, and what they believe affects what they do; that children are open to propaganda because they are unsuspecting; that the catchy tune is remembered a long time and the words of the commercial along with it; that receptivity changes with years of growing. The voice and diction of a political candidate with a repetition of phrases influence people and lull their sensibilities.

Some corporations have done a commendable job of combining their advertising with public service. Along with promoting specific products and services some have encouraged preservation of our forests, promoted better health, safer highways and citizen responsibility.

Encouraged by the fact that too many people were interested in "how much do I pay down" and "how much do I pay a month," without regard for the total cost of consumer goods or services, true interest rates have customarily been hidden by all who made this assessment. Title I of the Consumer Protection Act is the "truth in lending" provision which forces disclosure of true interest rates being charged the consumer. Requiring that the public be told all is a means of protection from high interest and from the desire to borrow heavily for a better life. "Truth in lending" helps because it translates devious mathematics into simple terms which most buyers or borrowers can understand. The consumer should be encouraged to weigh the personal value of paying such fees against the value of a cash purchase without a premium.

It is time that the profession publicly acknowledge its belief that the use of sugar is not good nutritional practice, and actively support the utilization of nutritious snacks in schools. It should also be active in promoting changes in misleading advertising of dentifrices and mouthwashes. Above all, it must practice what it preaches to patients, and set a good example for the public.

Challenge: Sex and Changing Attitudes

Sex and moral standards are probably more interesting to the general public than business or politics. The changes characterizing this era impose severe strains on the moral system. Sex is discussed more freely and frequently by more people today than ever before. Is there a core of moral values which can be maintained or must moral and ethical codes be adapted to these new conditions?

We see a swiftly changing definition of morality and a search for a more meaningful basis for ethical content in contemporary art, drama and literature. Obscenity, promiscuity and prostitution have commonly been considered as immoral, but today there seems to be a lack of uniform standards by which to judge conduct, books and pictures. Who is to make this judgment of material and its suitability for various age groups or classes of people? Is all questionable material to be outlawed or should the individual be educated to choose wisely? In banning a book, for instance, the risks of suppressing its ideas must be weighed against the risks of its being widely circulated to an impressionable audience.

Marriage and family relationships are undergoing change, but that does not mean that they will be discarded. Monogamy has proved to be the best way to help a child grow into a mature being within society. Saving the family structure will depend on an about-face in current mores which can mainly be brought about by the happily married. To understand marriage as a viable institution, young people need to see its value in their parents and other adults of the family. It will be this example of parents, and the preparation which they and schools can give young people, which will influence change.

Discussion of divorce, birth control, premarital and extramarital sex experience has mainly led to confusion and a need for real moral guidance. Even those assumed to be authorities are perplexed and offer conflicting advice. Seemingly a day of permissiveness has dawned and each group can impose standards on its own members, but not on all groups. Despite the fact that it is controversial in character, a broader and deeper knowledge of human sexuality is desirable and useful to most persons.

Conventions of morality in the past were more easily administered because of the way people lived, although there were imperfections even then. Traditionally mores have been flexible to the extent that female chastity was demanded (contradictorily prostitutes were accepted), but males were not bound by such precepts. One fact that should be considered is that chastity can be forfeited at any time, but once it is violated it is never recovered.

Sex is a physiological function as are walking and talking. Although young people today seem more mature, they need to learn that sex is incidental to an enduring partnership of marriage and home. Compatibility of partners is a process, not an accident, and couples must work at adaptation. Couples must learn that love can grow; it is not just here and gone, and with a firm foundation it has something to grow on and with.

Challenge: The Church and Government

Free-thinking individuals, seeking the right to worship as they pleased rather than by government decree, were the nucleus of America's first settlers from the Old World. It was because of the demands of social necessity that the United States was founded. There was proof in the lessons of their experiences that led these people to assert a distinct difference between church and state. Written in our Constitution as Article 1 is "Congress shall make no law respecting an establishment of religion or prohibiting the free exercise thereof . . . ."; thus, a pluralism was early established. Roger Williams feared that the state would corrupt the church, and Thomas Jefferson feared that the church would corrupt the state, but they were in agreement that the two should be separate.

The Christian ethic is basically one of love, implying social relationships. The Church is expected to contribute to the moral life of society and therefore presumably cannot shun issues such as segregation, poverty, greed and hypocrisy—all of which become involved with government. When prayers were banned in schools there was regret expressed at the government striking at a tradition. The United States has been essentially a religious nation, and freedom of religion is a sacred American heritage. The separation of church and state involves the question of federal aid to education. If the government financially supports church-controlled schools, then can it logically and morally have some control over school activities as it does over secular schools? Ethical teachings of all religions give us unattainable ideals useful in giving us absolute standards by which to judge personal and social righteousness. The Church today is facing significant implications in the stance it takes.

Challenge: Alienation of Students

Industrial capitalism has always been criticized, but it has been responsible for many advancements in methodology and in the labor force. There is still much to be desired, but improvements such as the reduction of the work week, the elimination of poverty for four-fifths of the American population, and the provision of education for all have been made. Ethnic prejudice spoils the record, but the opportunity is still available for those who are willing to earn it.

Without exaggerating achievements, or ignoring the impairment of growth, it is paradoxical that there is such widespread disillusionment among those who are not economically disadvantaged. It is not just the poverty and inequality which have apparently disillusioned them; it appears to be the whole way of life of modern society. It is a protest of people, mainly on our campuses, who feel, or at least say they do, that they are isolated, displaced and rootless.

Did the rebellious acts of the younger generation represent a personal failure with growing up in a complex society or were they symptoms of a real breakdown in society? Was such behavior purely exhibitionism or was it a valid moral criticism? The generation largely involved was raised by permissive parents and this was often their first confrontation with authority. During the depression years these parents struggled to reach a middle or upper-middle class existence; these young people went the other direction, from riches to rags. J. S. Mill long ago said "It is better to be a human being dissatisfied than a pig satisfied; better to be Socrates dissatisfied than a fool satisfied." Some might rather live like pigs than to live in a rat-race society, but it is difficult for the majority to accept what is to them a lower standard as a way of life.

The ranks of renegades from society included artists, writers, and teachers as well as students representing a new style of life. They declared that they were seeking honesty from artificial values. Middle-class values, possessions and conformity were discarded. These newly free creatures showed disdain for social position and material possessions, perhaps relishing their freedom and enjoying shocking their elders. They were against anything they thought diminished the value of the individual.

The questions they raised were profound but their solutions were unrealistic. They gave up social responsibility, they were dissatisfied with educational experiences. They were merely "against" things as they were.

Other groups were more militant and preferred rebellion to retreat from reality. They preached alienation from the "establishment" and resorted to demonstrations on civil rights, war or some current event. Although they were vague concerning real goals or programs, they were coercive and courageous in their protests.

Boys and girls dressed in identical clothes and affecting identical hair styles are in a sense telling us that secondary sex characteristics are not that important. Instead of fostering racial antagonisms, these young people are comfortably integrated, espousing problems of poverty, the ghetto and leisure. Instead of grasping at individual property or material possessions of any kind, they happily share. They take great pride in being able to do without "things." The new left-leaning liberal is not prepared to renounce private property but the radical, revolutionary socialist does not hold private property in esteem. Instead, he demands that it be shared for "the people." The traditional Pandora's box has been opened again letting out the radicals who are gadflies to society and to its institutions which must come to grips with the problems of today's people.

Unrest on college, and even high school, campuses has forced the question "Who's in charge?" and its corollary "Who should be in charge?" Should it be the trustees, the president, the faculty or the students? There is need to reexamine these various roles and offer more participation to all groups. Today's students are more mature than those of past years and are more perceptive critics of society. Keeping in mind that the student generation is four years in duration and that college and university personnel are more permanent, channels of communication ought to be opened to students who should be included in decision making. There should not be authoritarian leadership, but leadership should be decisive. The decisions made now will not only affect students but unprecedented numbers of people in significant ways.

The stated issues of organized, vocal groups of students can be real or can be disguises for such things as the destruction of our political and social systems as a whole. All change involves some conflict as well as cooperation between groups. Conflict should not, then, be abolished, but it must be given boundaries. The group must learn and believe that reform from within is preferable from moral and common sense viewpoints to tearing down established social structures—and then trying to rebuild on nothing.

To educate is to produce desirable changes in the student, changes which will make a difference in his life. The teacher's job is to teach, to challenge, to criticize and to evoke thought. The student needs to be stimulated, challenged to survive in the real world. Among other things, the student must be made to accept his future responsibilities. The form and structure of education are being questioned, but the framework itself, the environment and the institution, are there, ready for regeneration. True academic freedom is achieved by defending the rights of all.

The university students not heard from perhaps are pragmatists. They want change in society in order to transform American life into something better and they want careers that will enable them to contribute to this transformation.

Challenge: Drugs

The use of drugs is an ancient device to escape reality, not restricted to this generation or to youthful rebels. As a group, however, the young are the most vulnerable to experimentation with new products. Addictive drugs when not available to the user lead to crimes in order to obtain money for their purchase. Non-addictive drugs alter perception, affecting the mind with resultant poor judgment or hallucinations and can be psychologically habit forming.

Use of marijuana and LSD-25 (lysergic acid diethylamide) are not limited to fringe groups, for the conventional person looking for kicks is a susceptible prospect, too. The marijuana user is looking for euphoria, but "it can impair judgment and memory; it can cause anxiety, confusion or disorientation and it can induce temporary psychotic episodes in certain predisposed people" (President's Advisory Commission on Crime and Law Enforcement, February 1967, pp. 12-14). It also has a tendency to release inhibitions, the effect depending on the individual and the circumstances. Marijuana does not lead to heroin directly, but certainly predisposes by association with those who peddle illicit drugs.

The LSD user is often looking for understanding and self exploration, neither of which is honestly found by this means. Changes in sensation, particularly in vision, and other effects can be a state of anxiety or depression. Long-term usage results in organic brain changes. One of the chief dangers of LSD may be chromosome fragmentation, causing the same type of defects in babies as does the atom bomb.

Stimulants such as amphetamines cause brain and liver damage and deterioration of social, familial and moral values. They can easily become habituating. The sedatives and tranquilizers, barbiturates and meprobamate, reduce tension and anxiety but are addictive.

The risks inherent in the use of any of these drugs must be balanced against the mistaken notion of suppression of individual rights. Users argue that it is the individual's right to choose, to have a private experience which is not publicly sanctioned. In considering the reconciliation of individual rights and the public good, it is necessary to determine whether laws are enacted to be enforced, as expressions of ideals, or to encourage discretion.

Most authorities agree that an unsatisfactory family relationship between adults and adolescents is one factor which stimulates experimentation in the use of drugs. The dangerous side effects of drugs are ignored or discounted because they produce the wanted feelings of love and belonging which are not received at home. To be effective counsellors, individuals hoping to influence young people using drugs must not be hypocritical about their own use of legal drugs, such as smoking when there is evidence connecting it with cancer and other diseases.

Not too many drug users are aware of the possibility of losing their civil rights pending conviction of possession of drugs. These can include the right to vote; to own a gun; to run for public office; to be a licensed physician, dentist, lawyer, architect or pharmacist; to work for city, county or federal government; to hold any position for which a bond is required. Is the risk involved worth taking a chance with drugs?

Conclusions

More questions than answers to the challenges which have been proposed may seem to be unsatisfactory, but stimulating individual thought and choice is far better than the easy stereotyped response which the uninformed will grasp as a placebo and the intelligent will not accept unconditionally. The future holds choices for all. Will it be regression and an attempt to re-create a bygone society? Will it be dedication to maintain the status quo? Or will it be the creation of and adaptation to a new society with new values and new visions? Neither the primitive nor the rigid Victorian society will do for tomorrow. The average individual must learn to encourage diversity and to appreciate differences in the special accomplishments and potentials of individuals, and must show more tolerance, courage and commitment.

The decade of the seventies will surely bring solutions to some of the current problems and will just as surely bring new issues for consideration. America is in a critical period and there are significant decisions to be made, decisions which will affect all citizens. Policies must be established regarding developing nations and the more intimate challenges of poverty, power and environment must be faced. These problems are not likely to go away by themselves, nor will the others which are sure to emerge as society continues its metamorphosis. Man has stepped on the moon, but has neglected the many who stand on the earth.

Dental hygienists, then, must face these and other challenges of the world in which they live, and learn to make their own ethical decisions—decisions which will affect them personally, will stimulate their profession and will reach perhaps an even broader sphere of influence. The crises faced repre-

sent danger and opportunity; the turning point for dental hygienists must
be toward progress.

References

Girvetz, Harry K., ed.: *Contemporary Moral Issues,* 2nd ed. Belmont, Wadsworth
Publishing Co., Inc., 1968.
President's Advisory Commission on Crime and Law Enforcement. Washington,
February 1967, pages 12-14.

Appendix

Association Platform—Adopted October 1969

In order to promote and insure the excellence of the professional standards of the American Dental Hygienists' Association, strengthen the functioning of the Association, and assure optimum discharge of its responsibilities, the membership, trustees, and officers set forth the following platform—a declaration of principles:

Education:
 (1) To participate actively in developing and implementing standards to be used for selecting candidates for this health career.
 (2) To encourage the establishment of programs offering basic dental hygiene education and promote the continued improvement of existing programs.
 (3) To provide leadership and support for the establishment of dental hygiene programs in educational settings which offer courses acceptable for transfer to baccalaureate, master's, or doctoral degree curriculums.
 (4) To promote continuing education for continued improvement of dental hygiene services and for retention of dental hygienists in the manpower force.

Manpower:
 (1) To initiate studies of manpower needs required to insure quality dental hygiene services for all people and to engage in appropriate activities to help meet these needs.

Practice:
 (1) To participate actively in the advancement of dental hygiene

through the development and implementation of standards to be used in licensure and practice.

Research and Health Services:
(1) To promote the research necessary to enlarge the scientific basis of dental hygiene, foster the dissemination of scientific knowledge, and assist in applying this knowledge to dental hygiene practice.
(2) To support and participate in the activities of agencies dedicated to the improvement of health standards throughout the world.

Legislation:
(1) To propose and promote legislation designed to provide financial assistance to students and to educational programs that meet Association standards.
(2) To promote social, economic, health, and education legislation supporting the objectives of the profession.
(3) To provide equal opportunities in education, employment, and advancement in dental hygiene practice through support of appropriate legislation.
(4) To encourage and participate in studies designed to improve dental hygiene licensing legislation to insure optimal service to the public.

Constituent Association Information

Constituent	Date of Licensure*	Date Ass'n. Formed*	Current Number of Schools**	Date of Initiation***	Number of Licensed D.H.***
Alabama	1919	1932	0		1226
Alaska	1953	1964	0		32
Arizona	1947	1953	2	1969	505
Arkansas	1923	1955	1	1968	168
California	1921	1919	12	1918	4532
Southern California		1943			
Colorado	1919	1923	2	1962	1043
Connecticut	1916	1913	1	1913 (1949)†	2067
Delaware	1925	1932	0		200
District of Columbia	1924	1929	1	1934	507
Florida	1925	1926	5	1962	1900
Georgia	1927	1928	6	1967	1837
Hawaii	1920	1924	1	1961	447
Idaho	1950	1962	1	1961	109
Illinois	1945	1932	8	1922	891†††
Indiana	1945	1946	4	1950	439†††
Iowa	1921	1921	2	1953	527
Kansas	1935	1941	2	1966	466
Kentucky	1942	1953	3	1952	344

Constituent Association Information (Continued)

Constituent	Date of Licensure*	Date Ass'n. Formed*	Current Number of Schools**	Date of Initiation***	Number of Licensed D.H.***
uisiana	1929	1948	3	1960	315
ine	1917	1927	2	1961	318
ryland	1948	1954	3	1970	850
ssachusetts	1918	1922	5	1917	2043
chigan	1921	1921	8	1921	2601
nnesota	1919	1925	4	1921	1347
ssissippi	1928	1929	1	1970	70
ssouri	1947	1958	2	1951	700
ntana	1935	1963	1	1974††	100
braska	1949	1947	1	1964	182
vada	1947	1961	0		76
w Hampshire	1919	1919	1	1970	334
w Jersey	1948	1946	5	1948	1298
w Mexico	1951	1960	1	1961	168
w York	1916	1916	10	1916	7021†††
rth Carolina	1929	1948	7	1953	743
rth Dakota	1947	1968	1	1965	97
io	1920	1920	6	1945	1741
lahoma	1919	1956	2	1970	286
gon	1951	1952	5	1949	758
nnsylvania	1921	1923	5	1921	2512†††
ode Island	1931	1945	1	1960	220†††
th Carolina	1922	1953	2	1966	277
th Dakota	1939	1955	1	1967	118
nnessee	1920	1931	4	1927	677
xas	1950	1940	12	1955	1281
ah	1953	1949	0		90
rmont	1921	1956	1	1949	288
ginia	1950	1954	2	1967	557
shington	1921	1921	5	1950	992
st Virginia	1915	1925	3	1938	384†††
sconsin	1921	1926	3	1923	1346
oming	1921	1957	1	1969	82
rto Rico	1947	1972	1	1968	2†††

*Poll of Constituent Associations, 1971
*Accredited and accreditation eligible dental hygiene programs, Council on Dental Education, ADA, June 1974
*Requirements and Registration Data: Dental Hygiene 1974, Division of Educational Measurements, Council on Dental Education, ADA
Fones' school closed after three classes graduated. Reopened in 1949
Information not available left blank except Southern California. Those figures are included under California.
Projected date
1970 data

Chronology of the ADHA

1920   Discussion in Boston of forming national organization. Idea dropped.

1923   July: Dental Hygienists' Association of California and Dr. Guy S. Milberry presented resolution to ADA, requesting promotion of a national dental hygiene association.
September 12: American Dental Hygienists' Association organized in Cleveland, Ohio. Constitution and Bylaws provisionally accepted, officers elected. Dues $2. California, Colorado, Connecticut, Illinois, Iowa, Massachusetts, Michigan, New York, Ohio, Pennsylvania, West Virginia represented by forty-six dental hygienists.

1924   No meeting.

*1925   Winifred Hart. Louisville, Kentucky, 153 members. Constitution and Bylaws accepted. Honorary members elected.

1926   Edith Hardy Rector. Philadelphia, Pennsylvania. Journal established to begin January 1927. Code of Ethics approved.

1927   Ethel Covington. Detroit, Michigan. Dues raised to $3, 467 members. Association incorporated. Postgraduate course mentioned.

1928   Mildred Gilsdorf. Minneapolis, Minnesota. Official seal adopted. Constitution and Bylaws revised for incorporation. Dental hygienist on ADA Section program. Twelve schools, 2,000 total graduates.

1929   Charlotte Sullivan. Washington, D.C. Dental hygiene represented through communications on President Hoover's "Committee on Costs of Medical Care."

*1930   Cora Ueland. Denver, Colorado. President Ueland speaker for ADA program. Children's Dental Health Week mentioned.

*1931   Gladys S. Myers. Memphis, Tennessee. Thirty-one states licensed the dental hygienist. Nineteen constituent associations, sixteen schools. Official ADHA pin designed. Code of Ethics revised.

1932   Evelyn G. Wallace. Buffalo, New York. General members allowed to sit and listen to House of Delegates. Educational survey made. Twenty-three constituents, seventeen schools.

*1933   Helen B. Brown. Chicago, Illinois. Board of Trustees ex-officio members of House without vote. Journal to be quarterly starting in 1934. First verbatim minutes.

1934   A. Rebekah Fisk. St. Paul, Minnesota. Junior ADHA approved. Civil Service qualifications protested.

*Deceased

1935 Addibel F. Hall. New Orleans, Louisiana. Recommended "high school graduate" as one requirement for state licensure qualification; Civil Service employees be graduate dental hygienists. Curriculum survey report.

1936 Frances Shook. San Francisco, California. Trustees increased from six to nine. Scholarship Fund established.

1937 Margaret A. Bailey. Atlantic City, New Jersey. Bylaws revised.

1938 Agnes Morris Henry. St. Louis, Missouri. Survey of dental health programs initiated in states. Junior ADHA accepted. Recommended that all dental hygienists, graduates or not, be accepted as charter members by organizing states.
Dr. Fones died.

*1939 Helen Baukin. Milwaukee, Wisconsin. Education Committee surveyed duties, needs and remuneration of the dental hygienist. Suggested that all programs be minimum of two years.

1940 Cecilia P. Angel. Cleveland, Ohio. Fones' Loan Fund established.

1941 Dorothy O'Brien. Houston, Texas. Dental hygienists in armed services. Public Relations Committee to recruit students. War Service Committee.

1942 Boston, Massachusetts. Meeting cancelled due to World War II travel restrictions.

1943 Mary Zoepfel. Cincinnati, Ohio. Asked that dental hygienists be granted commissions in US Army. Northern and Southern California asked for two associations with one delegate. Nine trustee districts established. Past president member of Board for one year and given life membership. Urged that service-trained dental hygienists take recognized course when returning to civilian life.

1944 Isabell Kendrick. Chicago, Illinois. No scientific or social meetings. Committee appointed to work on standardization of training of dental hygienists.

1945 New York City. No general meeting because of World War II restrictions. Ad Interim Committee met.

1946 Margaret Jeffreys. Miami, Florida. France interested in dental hygienists. Dues raised to $5. Discussion of degree: should it be BS in Dental Hygiene or Health Education? Considered education and licensure of armed services personnel. Annual reports mimeographed and circulated instead of printed in *Journal*.

*Deceased

1947   Sophie Booth. Boston, Massachusetts. ADA House of Delegates adopted the Council on Dental Education Requirements for Accrediting of Schools for Dental Hygienists. Three schools offer BS with two years prior college, seven offer additional work and five give full credit. Bylaws revised.

*1948   Mabel McCarthy. Chicago, Illinois. Office of part-time executive secretary created. ADHA opposed to increase in field of practice until ADA indicates desire for dental hygienists to assume added duties. Several states allow fluoride application by dental hygienists. Forty-one states, District of Columbia, Hawaii and Puerto Rico licensed dental hygienists.

1949   Dr. Frances Stoll. San Francisco, California. Conference in Chicago on Teaching Programs for Training of Dental Hygienists. Met with ADA Council on Dental Education to help establish accreditation procedures. Proxy trustee at meeting. Membership recruitment letter from Central Office was first national effort.

1950   Evelyn E. Maas. Atlantic City, New Jersey. All US dental hygiene programs now two years. Forty-six states license the dental hygienist. Reference committees used. Topical fluoride approved.

1951   Blanche Downie. Washington, D.C. ADA Workshop discussed aims and objectives of dental hygiene education, curriculum needs, development of minimum standards and recommendations. All states licensed dental hygienists. All state constitutions were in conformity. Accreditation started in June. Aptitude test discussed.

1952   Betty Krippene. St. Louis, Missouri. Four schools accredited. Central Office reorganization committee.

1953   Evelyn Hannon. Cleveland, Ohio. Twenty-five schools accredited, four more scheduled. Dental hygiene employment, duties, remuneration were surveyed. University of Michigan Workshop. Code of Ethics revised.

1954   Laura Peck Fitch. Miami Beach, Florida. *Journal* cover redesigned. Disability Income Insurance offered. Dues to $7.

1955   Sarah Hill. San Francisco, California. California allowed one delegate for each constituent. Resume of annual session actions sent to Board, delegates and constituent associations.

1956   Marjorie Thornton. Atlantic City, New Jersey. Worked on upgrading Civil Service status of dental hygienist. Fluoridation of water supplies endorsed. Official constituent charters designed by Frances Shook.

1957   Dr. March Fong. Miami Beach, Florida. Educational Trust Fund established to accept grant funds from W. K. Kellogg Foundation to continue aptitude and achievement testing plans. Central Office to be moved to Chicago with full-time executive secretary, January 1958. House voted no membership restriction based on race, creed, color. "Needs of Central Office" Committee appointed. Board to meet two days before annual session rather than during session.

*1958   Beth Linn. Dallas, Texas. First Mid-Year Board Meeting. Parliamentarian employed on annual basis. National Board approved. Officers conference. Increase ADHA districts from nine to twelve.

1959   Helen Garvey. New York City. "Careers in Dental Hygiene" developed. Committee on Special Studies appointed.

1960   Tillie Ginsburg. Los Angeles, California. Office of third vice president eliminated. First speaker of the House of Delegates elected.

1961   Edna Bradbury. Philadelphia, Pennsylvania. Dues to $15. Constituent associations given proportional representation.

*1962   Anne Ragsdale, Miami Beach, Florida. First National Board examination for dental hygienists given. Four dental hygiene representatives on committee. International Dental Congress in Cologne, Germany, ADHA represented and dental hygienists presented clinics.

1963   Margaret S. Hunt. Atlantic City, New Jersey. Film on dental hygiene authorized.

1964   Janet R. Burnham. San Francisco, California. ADA, AADS, AADE, ADHA workshop discussed standards for dental hygiene education "Female" deleted from Bylaws.

1965   Irene Navarre. Las Vegas, Nevada. ADA, AADS, AADE, ADHA workshop, in-depth study of present and potential duties of dental hygienists. AADE liaison committee reactivated. Association evaluation by management consultant firm to review structure and function. Career film "A Bright Future" completed and premiered.

1966   Alberta Beat. Dallas, Texas. Central Office moved to new ADA building. Task Force Committee appointed to define dental hygiene expansion of services.

*Deceased

1967   Wilma Motley. Washington, D.C. Division of Educational Services established. ADHA sponsored workshop on standards and goals of certificate, baccalaureate and graduate programs in dental hygiene. Interagency Taskforce committee requested. L.R.P. goals presented.

1968   Wilma Motley. Miami Beach, Florida. Bylaws underwent major revision. Newsletter sent to all members. Operations and Procedures Manual approved. Legal definition of dental hygiene practice and revised principles of dental hygiene education accepted.

1969   Patricia McLean. New York City. Regional consultants to developing and established dental hygiene programs. Principles of Ethics revised. Association platform adopted. Clinical teachers institute held in Seattle, Washington. Washington representative appointed. Continuing education requirements endorsed. Admission requirements of all US and Canadian dental hygiene schools published in bound form.

1970   Lona Hulbush Jacobs. Las Vegas, Nevada. Dues to $25 on January 1, 1971; junior members $3. Trustee Workshop. Trustee district boundaries realigned. ADAA liaison committee appointed. Interagency Taskforce Committee appointed. First International Symposium on Dental Hygiene sponsored by ADHA in Italy. Operation and Procedures Manual distributed. "Curriculum Essentials" approved. Journal published bi-monthly.

1971   Kay Gandy. Atlantic City, New Jersey. Second Symposium in Switzerland. "Project Alliance" studied. Washington office opened and full-time representative authorized. Representation at F.D.I. meeting, Munich, Germany. All but three states and Puerto Rico accept National Board Dental Hygiene Examination.

1972   Diane McCain. San Francisco, California. Third Symposium in England. Multiple scientific sessions at annual meeting.

1973   Jeanne Fox. Houston, Texas. Bylaws completely revised. Fourth Symposium in Amsterdam. 50th Anniversary year.

1974   Konnetta Putman, Washington, D.C. COCD and Educational Assessment projects. Expansion of Central Office. Scopes Manual.

Address by Mrs. Wright to the Newly Formed American Dental Hygienists' Association, Cleveland, Ohio, September 12, 1923

Madam President, members of the American Association of Dental Hygienists.

I have been commissioned by the Council on Mouth Hygiene and Public Instruction of the American Dental Association to present to you on this occasion a gavel.

It is fitting that as your organization is kindred to that of the American Dental Association that you should have some bond from the older organization at this, your time of organization. Realizing that the conduct of your business in the future will demand some instrument of authority, this gavel has been chosen with the hope that in the deliberations of your body you may feel at all times that there is a kindred interest felt in you by the other organization.

This is a great occasion in the annals of hygienists. This is the birth of what will one day be a mighty organization. Pioneering in any profession is hard and rugged. It is the trying out time—the time that will build for a future depending on the strength or weakness manifest at this early stage. What nursing is to medicine, just so will the hygienist be to the dental profession. Can you imagine the surgeon or physician of today making a success of his profession without the assistance of the trained nurse? Just so the professions of hygienist and dentist are allied. The one is dependent on the other. There are certain marked lines for each to follow, certain circumscribed paths beyond which neither should stray, all leading to more effective service.

I feel it an honor that on this occasion I have been delegated to present you this gavel. I also feel honored that this instrument which is to be wielded at your meetings was fashioned from a stick of wood under my direction. It is patterned after the gavel that was used by Judge Taft at the Peace Conference. May it always be used peacefully, and may it be a mute witness of the development of a great profession that will have no backward tendencies, always going ahead and making a place for itself among the great professions of the world.

ANNA MIMS WRIGHT
(Mrs. Wm. R.)

Index

ABULCASIS, 81
Accreditation of schools, 116, 144, 146
Achievement test, dental hygiene, 145
Ad-Interim Committee, 117
Admission requirements, 144, 146
Allen, John, 19
American Association of Dental Examiners, 116, 144, 147, 149, 150
American Association of Dental Schools, 116, 144, 145, 147, 150
American Dental Assistants Association, 116, 150
American Dental Association, 19, 85, 111, 139, 142, 144, 145, 146, 147, 150
  civil defense and, 118
  conferences of, 116
  Council on Dental Education of, 116, 142, 144, 145, 150
  liaison with, 116
American Dental Hygienists' Association, administration of, 118
  annual sessions of, 116, 124
  Board of Trustees of, 123, 133
  Central Office of, 118–119
  chronology of, 174–178
  committees of, 123, 124, 135, 139, 141, 149, 150
  constituent associations of, 135, 172
  Constitution and Bylaws of, 111, 113, 121, 126
  educational programs of, 138
  executive secretary of, 118
  exhibits and clinics of, 114
  history of, 108
  House of Delegates of, 117, 122, 133

  incorporation of, 121
  membership of, 52, 121, 125, 126, 132, 148
  oath of, 115
  objectives of, 121
  officers of, 118, 123, 130, 133
  platform of, 171
  principles of ethics of, 20–21, 134
  publications of, 120, 123, 127, 128–130
  scholarships of, 102, 141
  structure and function of, 121–124
  Washington representative of, 138
American Dental Laboratory Association, 128
American Fund for Dental Health, 124, 144
American Journal of Dental Science, 85, 86
Andrews, Robert Robin, 87
Annual sessions, 116, 124
Aquinas, Thomas, 4
Aristotle, 13
Arnold, Benedict, 155
Ashurbanipal, 54
Assault, 72
Atkinson, C. B., 88
Avicenna, 81

BAKER, JOHN, 82
Ball, Louise C., 103
Barber surgeons, 79
Beatty, B. Elizabeth, 102
Board of Trustees, 123, 133
  districts and, 134
  reports of, 117
  workshop and, 118

CKKD